Respiratory Guidelines

(Asthma and COPD)

for

Family Practice

2nd Edition

Respiratory Review Panel

➢ *Peer-reviewed*

➢ *Evidence-based*

➢ *User-friendly*

This independent initiative is supported entirely through purchases of the guideline. All proceeds will be directed to maintaining and updating the guidelines.

To purchase copies
please visit our website or e-mail, write, call, or fax:

www.mumshealth.com

guidelines@mumshealth.com

MUMS GUIDELINES CLEARINGHOUSE

Suite 901 – 790 Bay St.,
Toronto ON M5G 1N8

Telephone: (416) 597-6867
Fax: (416) 597-8574

Check our website for possible corrections to the document and discounts offered on our publications.

Comment sheets are provided at the end of the document and at www.mumshealth.com.

Library and Archives Canada Cataloguing in Publication

Respiratory (Asthma and COPD) Guidelines for Family Practice/Respiratory Review Panel. -- 2nd Ed.

Originally published under the following title: Guidelines for the treatment of chronic obstructive pulmonary disease (COPD).

Includes biographical references.

ISBN 1-894332-06-7

1. Lungs--Diseases, Obstructive--Treatment. 2. Lungs--Diseases, Obstructive--Diagnosis I. Respiratory Review Panel II. MUMS Guideline Clearinghouse

RC776.O3G85 2007   616.2'4   C2006-903698-5

While great effort has been taken to assure the accuracy of the information, the Canadian Respiratory Review Panel, publisher, printer, and others contributing to the preparation of this document cannot accept liability for errors, omissions, or any consequences arising from the use of the information. Since this document is not intended to replace other prescribing information, physicians are urged to consult the manufacturers and other available drug information literature before prescribing.

Table of Contents

Cont'd

The Canadian Respiratory Review Panel

Meyer Balter
Respiratory Medicine
Toronto ON

Charles Bayliff
Pharmacy
London ON

Francine Borduas
Family Medicine
Neufchatel QC

Andrew Braude
Respiratory Medicine
North York ON

Carol Bruce
Family Medicine
Carp ON

Kenneth Chapman
Respiratory Medicine
Toronto ON

Lisa Cicutto
Nursing
Toronto ON

Donald Cockcroft
Respiratory Medicine
Saskatoon SK

Robert Cowie
Respiratory Medicine
Calgary AB

Ian Crawford
Family Medicine
Kingston ON

Anthony D'Urzo
Family Medicine
Toronto ON

Mark Fitzgerald
Respiratory Medicine
Vancouver BC

Paul Hernandez
Respiratory Medicine
Halifax NS

Richard Hodder
Respiratory Medicine
Ottawa ON

Robert Hyland
Respiratory Medicine
Toronto ON

Lawrence Jackson
Pharmacy
Toronto ON

Brent Jensen
Pharmacy
Saskatoon SK

Alan Kaplan
Family Medicine
Richmond Hill ON

John Jordan
Family Medicine
London ON

Josiah Lowry
Family Medicine
Orillia ON

Bernard Marlow
Family Medicine
Toronto ON

Frank Martino
Family Medicine
Brampton ON

Andrew McIvor
Respiratory Medicine
Hamilton ON

James Meuser
Family Medicine
Toronto ON

Denis O'Donnell
Respiratory Medicine
Kingston ON

Tom Perry
Clinical Pharmacology
Vancouver BC

Paolo Renzi
Respiratory Medicine
Montreal QC

Walter Rosser
Family Medicine
Kingston ON

John I. Stewart
Family Medicine
Port Perry ON

Charlene Welsh
Nursing
Toronto ON

Scientific/Editorial Staff

Jason Aldred, BScPhm

Elise Balaisis, BScH

Mirjana Chionglo, BScPhm

Laurie Dunn, MSc, BScPhm

Daniella Gallo, BScPhm, PharmD

Valentina Jelincic, BScPhm

Evan H. Kwong, MSc, BSc(Pharm)

Alex McLellan, BScPhm

Amita Patel, BScPhm, PharmD

John Pilla, MSc, BScPhm

Fariba Rahbary, BScPhm, PharmD

Loren Regier, BSP, BA

Simone R. Singh, Hon BSc

Serena Verma, MD, BSc(Pharm)

Guideline Reviewers (1998 - 2006)

Many thanks to the individuals below who took part in the review process in the 1998 guidelines and over the course of the past 8 years. We greatly appreciate your support.

Charlie Bayliff
Pharmacy
London ON

Neil Bell
Family Medicine
Edmonton AB

Lynne Benjamin
Family Medicine
Oakville ON

Norman Bottum
Family Medicine
Haliburton ON

Jean Bourbeau
Respiratory Medicine
Montreal QC

Joseph Braidy
Respiratory Medicine
Montreal QC

Cindy Breitkreutz
Family Medicine
Whitehorse YK

Paul Chabun
Family Medicine
Hazelton BC

Richard Coutts
Family Medicine
Midland ON

Peter Daniel
Family Medicine
Orillia ON

Peter Deimling
Family Medicine
Orillia ON

Lisa Dolovich
Pharmacy
Hamilton ON

Neil Donen
CME/Family Medicine
Victoria BC

Anthony D'Urzo
Family Medicine
Toronto ON

Geordie Fallis
Family Medicine
Toronto ON

Syd Feldman
Family Medicine
Willowdale ON

Norman Flett
Family Medicine
Dundas ON

Christopher Frank
Family Medicine
- Geriatrics
Kingston ON

Michael Gilman
Family Medicine
Toronto ON

Roger Goldstein
Respiratory Medicine
Toronto ON

Ronald Grossman
Respiratory Medicine
Mississauga ON

Vonda Hayes
Family Medicine
Halifax NS

G.H. Jonat
Family Medicine
Saskatoon SK

Jane Lindsay
Pulmonary Rehabilitation
Kitchener ON

Lianne McFarlane
Pharmacy
Dartmouth NS

Bruce McLeod
Emergency Medicine
Port Williams NS

J.S. McMillan
Family Medicine
Regina SK

Stephen McMurray
Family Medicine
Brockville ON

James Meuser
Family Medicine
Toronto ON

Ken Ng
Family Medicine
Markham ON

Nick Pimlott
Family Medicine
Toronto ON

Wayne Putnam
Family Medicine
Halifax NS

Lorne Rabuka
Family Medicine
Prince Albert SK

Tony Reid
Family Medicine
Orillia ON

Susan Ridout
Family Medicine
St. John's NF

Cathy Risdon
Family Medicine
Hamilton ON

James Ruderman
Family Medicine
Toronto ON

Brent Schneider
Pharmacy
Kingston ON

Stephen Shafran
Infectious Diseases
Edmonton AB

Dominick Shelton
Emergency Medicine
Toronto ON

G.W. Spiller
Family Medicine
Vernon BC

David Stubbing
Respiratory Medicine
Hamilton ON

Gabriel Thomasse
Family Medicine
Prince Albert SK

Irene Turpie
Geriatric Medicine
Hamilton ON

Peter Vaughan
Family Medicine
Guelph ON

Marvin Waxman
Family Medicine
Toronto ON

Deanna Williams
Pharmacy
Toronto ON

Preface

These guidelines are intended to meet the needs of busy community-based health practitioners who need concise, valid and clinically relevant advice that may assist them in the diagnosis and management of individuals with asthma and chronic obstructive pulmonary disease.

The guideline development process (known as PGD) is described in detail on the following page. This process combined with the balanced composition of the panel (e.g., specialists, family physicians, pharmacists, nurses, asthma educators, etc.) and independent funding is instrumental in limiting the different types of bias including competing or conflicting interests.

The panel hopes that these guidelines will help promote the best practice of medicine, including the most appropriate use of medications. They are not intended to replace a physician's judgment and are sufficiently flexible to allow health practitioners and patients to exercise judgement when choosing among available options.

Maintaining updated clinical guidelines requires the active, ongoing participation of physicians and interested groups. We ask for your assistance to keep these guidelines current and relevant to everyday clinical practice. Please send us your suggestions and recommendations using the **comment page at the back of the booklet or online at http://www.mumshealth.com.**

Use of the Guidelines

General

The drugs of choice in these guidelines were selected based on demonstrated efficacy, safety, clinical experience, potential drug interactions with concurrent medication, and anticipated patient compliance.

Dosage/Dosage Form

Dosage suggestions are in accord with accepted standards. In some instances, patients may require dosages in excess of monograph recommendations. Physicians are advised to consult the product monograph and other sources for additional information on age- and condition-specific dosing. This is particularly important with new or infrequently used drugs.

Prices/Costs

An **approximate daily** treatment cost for adults has been included for each drug, not including a professional dispensing fee or mark-up. Daily costs were derived based on the lowest priced interchangeable product as listed in the Ontario Drug Benefit Formulary (39th edition, 2006). If no listing was found, the manufacturers' price lists were consulted. The acquisition price will vary according to individual pharmacy practices; thus the estimated daily cost may not reflect all community situations.

The Peer-Reviewed Guideline Development (PGD) Process (1st and 2nd edition)

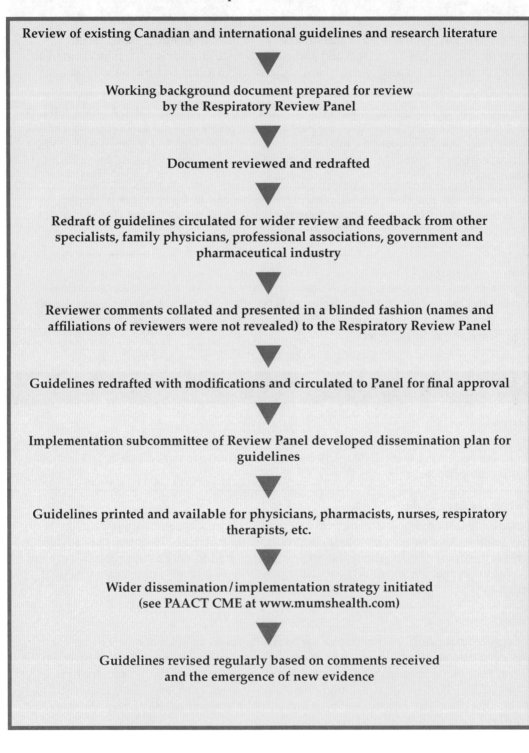

Review of existing Canadian and international guidelines and research literature

▼

Working background document prepared for review
by the Respiratory Review Panel

▼

Document reviewed and redrafted

▼

Redraft of guidelines circulated for wider review and feedback from other
specialists, family physicians, professional associations, government and
pharmaceutical industry

▼

Reviewer comments collated and presented in a blinded fashion (names and
affiliations of reviewers were not revealed) to the Respiratory Review Panel

▼

Guidelines redrafted with modifications and circulated to Panel for final approval

▼

Implementation subcommittee of Review Panel developed dissemination plan for
guidelines

▼

Guidelines printed and available for physicians, pharmacists, nurses, respiratory
therapists, etc.

▼

Wider dissemination/implementation strategy initiated
(see PAACT CME at www.mumshealth.com)

▼

Guidelines revised regularly based on comments received
and the emergence of new evidence

ASTHMA

OVERVIEW: General Characteristics of Asthma

Age of Onset	• Any age, usually < 40 years • Symptoms often first appear in childhood
Role of Smoking	• Not directly related but accelerates decline in lung function • Smoking adversely affects the condition and response to therapy • Maternal smoking increases the likelihood of wheezing in childhood • Consider second-hand smoke
History of Allergy/ Rhinitis	• Majority of patients with asthma have rhinitis and many individuals with persistent rhinitis (up to 30%) have or develop asthma (GINA 2006) • 70-90% of children with asthma may have allergies (AAAAI 2004) • Aspirin sensitivity triad (ASA intolerance, nasal polyps, rhinitis) can be associated with asthma and usually seen in patients over 40 years old
Family History	• Yes, a risk factor for asthma is parental history of asthma or eczema
Symptoms	• Wheezing, chest tightness, dyspnea, cough, and infrequent sputum production • Intermittent, variable, often paroxysmal and provoked by allergic or non-allergic stimuli (e.g., cold air, irritants, viral infections) • Frequently occur or worsen at night, awakening the patient • Exercise-induced bronchoconstriction may occur
Disease Course	• Usually stable with exacerbations
Spirometry	• Key element in diagnosis in older asthmatics (not usually reliable in children under the age of 6 years) • Useful to confirm an adequate response to therapy
Reversibility of Airflow Obstruction	• Airflow obstruction is usually episodic and completely reversible with therapy • FEV_1 is usually normal between attacks and improves quickly with bronchodilators • Normal FEV_1 may not be achievable in long-standing asthma, especially if poorly controlled
Hypoxemia	• Unusual; episodic with severe attacks
Chest X-ray	• Usually normal except during acute attacks (not usually required)

OVERVIEW: Management of Asthma

Prevention	• Control of allergens/triggers • Smoking cessation, Immunization
Non-pharmacological Therapy	• Education • Self-monitoring • Environmental control and trigger/allergen avoidance
Response to Therapy as Measured by Spirometry and Symptoms	• Marked improvement in spirometry with use of bronchodilators and steroids, or transient worsening with provocative testing (methacholine) • Goal is no symptoms, full activity
Pharmacotherapy (Treatment options for reaching acceptable asthma control)	1) SABA as needed for intermittent symptoms (always available as rescue medication and for preventing exercise-induced symptoms) 2) ICS (start with low dose) 3) Continue with ICS (low to moderate dose) and then add therapy with LABA (or next choice is LTRA or third choice is theophylline) 4) ICS (high doses) with LABA 5) In severe asthma addition of oral prednisone may be needed 6) Consider Anti-IgE therapy for patients with severe recalcitrant asthma with an allergic component (specialist supervision)
Adjunctive Therapy	• Topical nasal corticosteroid therapy can be used for rhinitis and nasal polyps
Acute Exacerbations (moderate to severe)	• SABA • Systemic corticosteroids • Inhaled anticholinergics added to SABA in moderate to severe exacerbations • Oxygen supplementation as needed

Legend	
SABA	Short-Acting Inhaled β_2-agonists (e.g., fenoterol, salbutamol, terbutaline). The formoterol fumarate dihydrate (Oxeze®) preparation is a long-acting inhaled β_2-agonists (LABA) that exhibits a rapid or fast onset of action and has been referred to as RABA (rapid-acting inhaled β_2-agonist) and FABA (fast-acting inhaled β_2-agonist) (Tattersfield 2001, Astra Product monograph). In asthma patients, ONLY Oxeze® (formoterol fumarate dihydrate) has been approved for rescue therapy and prevention of exercise-symptoms, and not Foradil® (formoterol fumarate). See product monograph for age-specific indications and dosing.
ICS	Inhaled Corticosteroid (e.g., beclomethasone, budesonide, ciclesonide, fluticasone)
LABA	Long-Acting Inhaled β_2-agonists (e.g., formoterol, salmeterol)
LTRA	Leukotriene Receptor Antagonist (e.g., montelukast, zafirlukast)
Anti - IgE	IgE monoclonal antibodies (e.g., omalizumab)

Background

Definition

"Asthma is characterized by paroxysmal or persistent symptoms such as dyspnea, chest tightness, wheezing, sputum production and cough, associated with variable airflow limitation and airway hyper-responsiveness to endogenous and exogenous stimuli. Inflammation and resultant effects on airway structure are considered to be the main mechanisms leading to the development and persistence of asthma." (Boulet 1999; Lemière 2004; NACTF 2000; NAEPP 1997).

Mortality/Morbidity

Between 1970 and 1984, illness and death from asthma increased by over 50% among Canadians 15 to 34 years of age (Mao 1987). Since 1987 asthma death rates have decreased in most age groups, with the highest rates persisting in those 65 years of age and older (CIHI 2001). Overall, death from asthma is uncommon and the rates are low compared to COPD.

Prevalence

Asthma has been noted as the most common chronic respiratory illness in North America (Boulet 1994). In Canada, the National Population Health Survey (NPHS) from 1998/99 indicated an overall 8.4% prevalence for physician-diagnosed asthma: 7.5% among adults (1.6 million) and 10.7% among children and teens (850,000). The prevalence was higher in young boys than in girls, whereas adult women were affected more often than men. The majority of individuals with current asthma reported frequent asthma symptoms (wheezing, shortness of breath or fatigue) either daily (14%) or several times a month (37%). In addition, 56% reported an asthma exacerbation in the past 12 months (CIHI 2001). Recent publications have documented similar prevalence rates (ICES 2006; Prodigy 2006) and an international report (GINA 2006) has noted that the prevalence across different countries ranges from 1% to 18% of the population. It was acknowledged that the lack of a precise and universally accepted definition of asthma makes reliable comparisons problematic.

Health Care Services and Costs

The 1996/97 NPHS Survey noted that 43% of individuals with current asthma visited their physicians 1 to 3 times in the previous year and 17% visited 4 or more times. Also, 18% had visited an emergency department at least once in the past year and 5.3% required hospital admission. The rates were highest in children under 5 years of age and in P.E.I., New Brunswick and Saskatchewan. However, hospitalization rates have been decreasing since 1987 and may reflect better disease control (CIHI 2001). In Canada, 20-25% of all childhood asthma exacerbations requiring hospitalization occur in September. During this time of the year, there may be an association with increased respiratory viruses and/or decreased use of anti-inflammatory medications (Johnston 2001, 2005).

Among current asthmatics, 22% experience restriction of daily activities for 1-5 days/year, while 13% are affected > 5 days/year (CIHI 2001). The cost of workdays lost annually because of asthma reached approximately $1 million dollars in 1987 and 1988 (Boulet 1994). A conservative estimate of total asthma costs in Canada in 1990 was $504 million dollars, of which drug costs were the largest component (Krahn 1996).

PART I
Diagnosis of Asthma

Diagnosis of Asthma in Children

Table 1. Diagnosis of Childhood (< 6 yrs) Asthma
(Becker 2005, GINA 2006)

Diagnosis of asthma in children (< 6 years) is primarily based on clinical judgement and an assessment of symptoms, history and physical findings

In children under 3 years of age neither lung function tests nor assessment of airway inflammation is helpful clinically.

Criteria supporting a diagnosis of asthma (likelihood of asthma increases as more criteria are met):

- Severe episode of wheezing/dyspnea
- Wheezing or dyspnea after 1 year of age
- 3 or more episodes of wheezing
- Chronic cough, especially at night or exercise-induced
- Clinical benefits from asthma medications (SABA, ICS)*
- Family history of atopy or asthma
- Personal history of atopy

*Note: Support for a diagnosis of asthma exists when a significant clinical improvement occurs during drug therapy and is followed by deterioration after therapy is discontinued.

Table 2. Differential Diagnosis of Wheezing in Children
(AAAAI 2004; Becker 2005; GINA 2006)

In most children (< 6 years), wheezing episodes are associated with viral respiratory illness

The respiratory syncytial virus (RSV) usually affects children < 2 years, whereas rhinovirus affects older children (2-6 years). The younger the child, the greater likelihood that a diagnosis other than asthma may explain recurrent wheezes. Wheezing does not always mean asthma, while asthma may be present without wheeze.

Differential diagnosis of wheezing in children:

- Allergy
- Aspiration
- Asthma
- Bronchiolitis
- Bronchopulmonary dysplasia
- Congenital anomalies/disease e.g., heart, intrathoracic
- Cystic fibrosis
- Foreign body aspiration
- Gastroesophageal reflux
- Immune system disorders
- Pertussis
- Primary ciliary dyskinesia syndrome
- Recurrent viral lower respiratory infections
- Rhinitis/sinusitis (chronic)
- Tuberculosis

Diagnosis of Asthma in Children (continued)

Table 3. Categories/Evolution of Wheezing
(Becker 2005, GINA 2006)

Among children (< 6 years) with wheezing, <u>50-60% outgrow the problem</u> (although it may reappear in adulthood). This percentage may include children originally mislabeled as "asthmatic"

Transient early-onset	Persistent early-onset	Persistent late-onset
Wheezing before 3 years of age which is often outgrown in the first 3 years. Often associated with prematurity and/or parental smoking.	Wheezing before 3 years of age and persists through school age and still present at age 12 in a large proportion. Typically have recurrent episodes of wheezing associated with acute viral respiratory infections, no evidence of atopy and no family history of atopy.	Wheezing usually after 3 years of age and less likely to resolve and often persists into adulthood. Typically have an atopic background, often with eczema and airway pathology that is characteristic of asthma.

Table 4. Role of Atopy (Allergy) in Persistent Asthma
(Becker 2005; Castro-Rodríguez 2000)

Recurrent wheezing in NON-ATOPIC children (< 6 years) is likely to resolve. However, ATOPY is a predictor of persistent asthma.

The following clinical index may help predict which wheezing child is more likely to experience persistent asthma into later childhood (6-13 years)

Stringent index	Loose index
Three or more episodes of wheeze during the first 3 years of life	**Any wheezing** during the first 3 years of life
PLUS either of:	**PLUS** either of:
At least 1 of the major risk factors (i.e., parental history of asthma or eczema)	At least 1 of the major risk factors (i.e., parental history of asthma or eczema)
OR	**OR**
At least 2 of 3 minor risk factors (i.e., eosinophilia, wheezing without colds, allergic rhinitis)	At least 2 of 3 minor risk factors (i.e., eosinophilia, wheezing without colds, allergic rhinitis)

Eosinophilia was considered to be present if eosinophils were $\geq 4\%$ of total white blood cells.

Physicians should obtain a personal and family history of atopy and look especially for the presence of atopic dermatitis during physical examination. The presence of atopy can be established by skin-prick testing or measurement of specific IgE antibodies and is suggested by elevated peripheral total IgE and blood eosinophils.

Diagnosis of Asthma in Older Children and Adults

Diagnosis of asthma is generally based on clinical findings and spirometry. **The usual symptoms of asthma include: wheezing, chest tightness, dyspnea, and cough.** These symptoms are variable, often paroxysmal and provoked by allergic or non-allergic stimuli (e.g., cold air, irritants, viral infections). The symptoms may occur or worsen at night, awakening the patient. Exercise-induced bronchospasm may also occur.

Pre- and post-bronchodilator spirometry can help identify a reversible component of airflow obstruction ($\geq 12\%$ of baseline and $\geq 200\,mL$ change in FEV_1), supporting a diagnosis of asthma while differentiating it from COPD. Spirometry is also useful to confirm an adequate response to therapy. See Appendix A and B for further information on measurements of lung function and tests for diagnosing and monitoring asthma.

Symptoms of asthma may be non-specific and thus ruling out other diagnoses is important. (Table 5).

Table 5. Differential Diagnosis for Asthma
(BTS 2005; GINA 2006; ICSI 2005)

Upper airway disease
- Rhinitis and sinusitis

Obstruction involving large airways
- Bronchiectasis from various causes, including cystic fibrosis
- Enlarged lymph nodes or tumour (benign or malignant)
- Foreign body in trachea or bronchus
- Laryngotracheomalacia, tracheal stenosis or bronchostenosis
- Post nasal drip
- Vocal cord dysfunction or laryngospasm
- Vascular rings or laryngeal webs

Obstruction of small airways
- Bronchopulmonary dysplasia
- COPD
- Cystic fibrosis
- Pulmonary infiltrates with eosinophilia
- Viral bronchiolitis or obliterative bronchiolitis

Other causes of respiratory symptoms
- Anxiety hyperventilation
- Aspiration from swallowing mechanism dysfunction
- Congestive heart failure
- Cough secondary to drugs
- Gastroesophageal reflux disease
- Pulmonary embolism
- Recurrent cough not due to asthma
- Sleep apnea

Factors Associated with Asthma

Allergens/Allergies (Almqvist 2003; Becker 2005; Brussee 2005; Caledon 2002; Gern 2004; GINA 2006; Melen 2001; Ownby 2002; Platts-Mills 2001; Wang 2005)	• Sensitization to cat/dog dander, dust mites allergens, and *Aspergillus* mould are independent risk factors for asthma-like symptoms up to 3 years of age. • Exposure to domestic dust mite and cat allergens during infancy may lead to sensitization at 4 years of age and, in case of cat allergens, to persistent wheeze. However, some epidemiologic studies suggest early childhood exposure to dogs and cats may protect against later sensitization. The issue remains controversial. • In infants with a family history of asthma and atopy, the initial development of asthma may be preventable by avoiding exposure to passive smoking and to allergens such as dust mites, cats, and cockroaches. • There may be an association between food sensitization and asthma.
Antibiotics (Johnson 2005; Marra 2006)	• Antibiotic use in early life may increase risk for atopy and asthma in children.
Diet (Friedman 2005; Devereux 2005)	• Some data suggest that infants fed formulas of cow's milk or soy protein have a higher incidence of wheezing in early childhood compared to breast fed infants. Also a suggestion that Western diets (containing more processed foods and margarine and less anti-oxidants and n-3 polyunsaturated fatty-acid) have contributed to the increase in asthma and atopic disease.
Exposure to Occupational Substances (For more information about occupational asthma and workplace sensitizers, see Appendix C) (GINA 2006; Newman 2004; Tarlo 1998))	• Estimated to account for 9-15% of adult-onset asthma. • If new-onset asthma develops during a person's working life, an occupational cause should be suspected and a detailed occupational history should be obtained. • Patient histories have been found to have high sensitivity but low specificity for diagnosis of occupational asthma. • Occupational asthma (irritant-induced or sensitizer-induced) should be differentiated from aggravation of pre-existing or coincidental asthma. • Objective investigations (e.g., serial PEF, challenge testing) are useful to confirm a diagnosis of occupational asthma. • It is recommended that the patient be referred early to a respirologist for formal documentation while still employed.
Family History (GINA 2006)	• Family history of allergy or asthma is associated with persistence or continuation of asthma through childhood.
Gender (GINA 2006)	• Before the age of 14 years, the prevalence of asthma in males in nearly twice that of girls. However, this pattern changes and by adulthood the prevalence is greater in women.
Obesity (Bergeron 2005; Beuther 2005, 2006; Brisbon 2005; Fantuzzi 2005; Ford 2005; Lucas 2005; Shore 2005; Sood 2005)	• Higher incidence and prevalence of asthma in obese adults and children. • Asthma may contribute to a sedentary lifestyle and obesity, but obesity has also been shown to be a risk factor and precede asthma. • Obesity may be a product of lifestyle changes in both diet and physical activity. Weight loss in obese individuals improves overall lung function and asthma symptoms, and reduces the use of asthma medications.
Tobacco Smoke (GINA 2006)	• Perinatal exposure to passive smoke is associated with a greater risk of developing asthma-like symptoms in early childhood. Tobacco smoking is associated with accelerated decline of lung function in people with asthma and may reduce response to drug therapy and overall asthma control.

When to Consider a Referral to a Specialist/Asthma Clinic

(For asthma clinics see: Asthma Society of Canada at www.asthma.ca; Canadian Lung Association at www.lung.ca) (BTS 2005; GINA 2006; ICSI 2005; NAEPP 1997, 2000)

- **Atypical presentation**

- **Severe persistent asthma**

- **A recent visit to the emergency department** due to an asthma exacerbation

- **Not meeting the goals of asthma therapy** after 3 to 6 months of treatment

- Physician concludes that the **patient is unresponsive to therapy**

- **Abnormal spirometry despite maximal or optimal therapy**

- **Requires prolonged oral or high-dose inhaled corticosteroids or has been treated with more than one courses of oral corticosteroids in the past year**

- **Co-morbid illnesses affect presentation and management** (e.g., sinusitis, nasal polyps, aspergillosis, severe rhinitis, vocal cord dysfunction, gastroesophageal reflux, chronic obstructive pulmonary disease)

- **Multiple diagnostic tests are indicated** (e.g., allergy skin testing, rhinoscopy, complete pulmonary function studies, provocative challenge, bronchoscopy)

- **Requires additional or specific education and counseling or training** on disease, treatment, and prevention (medication, self management, action plans, PEF)

- **Candidate for immunotherapy**

- **Under age 3 and requires care for moderate to severe asthma**

- **Occupational, environmental inhalant, or ingested substances are suspected** in provoking or contributing to symptoms

PART II
Management of Asthma

Asthma Management: Goals and Objectives

The overall goal is to improve health status and quality of life of the patient, as well as to reduce hospitalizations, morbidity, and premature mortality.

Symptoms of asthma are almost always reversible and preventable. A practical approach to management includes:

- Non-pharmacological approaches (education, self-monitoring)
- Smoking cessation (and elimination of exposure to second-hand smoke)
- Immunization
- Control of allergens / triggers
- Pharmacological therapy

Asthma Management: Checklist

- ☐ Identify **asthma allergens/triggers** (e.g., environmental, medications, etc.) and avoidance strategies

- ☐ Advise patient on benefits of **smoking cessation** and/or minimization of **exposure to passive smoke** and establish a strategy to quit

- ☐ Develop and educate patient on the use of an **asthma action plan**

- ☐ **Educate** patient (and parents of children) **about illness and medication**
  - Symptom recognition and evaluation
  - Purpose of medication
  - Possible adverse drug effects and how to minimize them

- ☐ Review **proper inhalation** technique

- ☐ Counsel patient on benefits vs. risks of **influenza vaccination**

- ☐ Advise females regarding special issues surrounding **pregnancy**
  - Minimization of exposure to triggers
  - Safety of asthma medication
  - Consequences of poor control for mother and fetus

- ☐ Review individual risk factors for osteoporosis in **elderly patients** and **post-menopausal females**, consider:
  - Preventative treatment
  - Osteoporotic treatment

- ☐ Consider **compliance**, **inhalation technique**, and **allergen avoidance** before making changes to treatment regimen in patients with sub-optimal control

- ☐ Emphasize that **asthma is a chronic disease that requires regular follow-up**

Non-pharmacological Approaches in Asthma
(Becker 2005; Boulet 1999, 2001; NACTF 2000)

Education

Education is integral for successful management of asthma, and should be provided to all patients. It may be of particular benefit to patients with high asthma-related morbidity or severe asthma and during visits to the emergency department and admissions to the hospital.

Allergen and trigger avoidance measures must be reinforced at regular intervals (see Table 7).

Patient self-monitoring using PEF or symptom frequency can be effective. The use of PEF as a self-monitoring tool may be useful in children or in asthmatics who are poor perceivers of airflow obstruction. However, no study has shown improved outcomes with PEF monitoring and compliance has been shown to be poor.

A **written action plan** for guided self-management should be developed for all patients. An action plan based on symptoms and use of the "stoplight" analogy is recommended. The plan provides patients with recommendations for medication use in the event of an increase in the severity or frequency of symptoms, or an increase in as needed bronchodilator, and/or a change in PEF, and when to seek medical attention.

Patients should be taught **how to properly use inhalational devices;** techniques should be checked at first use and periodically thereafter.

The approach to **pediatric asthma education** is not as clearly established. Beneficial effects have been observed in adolescents using education provided by peers.

Table 6. Prevention: Smoking Cessation and Immunization

Smoking Cessation	• Asthma patients who smoke have a poorer response to asthma medications (Pederson 1996; Chalmers 2002; Chaudhuri 2003) and should be encouraged to adopt strategies to stop smoking • A study found that asthma patients who stopped smoking experienced an improvement in their lung function (Chaudhuri 2006) • Minimizing or eliminating exposure to passive smoking is also important
Immunization	• Patients with asthma are at risk of influenza-related complications and annual influenza vaccination is recommended (Canadian Immunization Guide 2002) • There is limited/poor evidence to support routine pneumococcal vaccination in asthmatics (Shiekh 2004) and it is not currently recommended (Canadian Immunization Guide 2002)

Table 7. Prevention: Control of Allergens/Triggers
(AAAAI 2004; Boulet 1999, 2001; NACTF 2000; NAEPP 1997, 2002)

Colds or chest infections, exercise, tobacco smoke, pollen/grass/flowers, and dust are the most common triggers among asthmatics in Canada. Reduce or eliminate exposure to triggers:

Respiratory Infections	• To prevent respiratory infections in young children: promote good nutrition, avoid overcrowded daycare centres, institute infection-control procedures at daycare centres and consider influenza immunization
Tobacco Smoke	• Counsel patients and their household contacts on the benefits of smoking cessation • Discuss ways to create a smoke-free environment for the patient • Minimize exposure to second-hand smoke
Pollens (from trees, grass or weeds) and Outdoor Mould	• Minimize exposure during months that outdoor allergens are problematic
Indoor Mould	• Fix all leaks and eliminate water sources associated with mould growth • Attempt to keep indoor humidity at less than 50%
Indoor/Outdoor Pollutants and Irritants	• Minimize exposures to harmful agents in the home/workplace: wood-burning stoves or fireplaces, unvented stoves or heaters, other irritants (e.g., cleaning agents, sprays) • Use proper personal protective equipment in the workplace
Animal Dander (allergy tests)	• Remove animals from home or keep animals out of patient's room; air ducts should be covered with a dense filter (HEPA air cleaner); vacuum frequently
House Dust Mites	Essential: • Encase mattress in an allergen-impermeable cover; encase pillow in an allergen-impermeable cover or wash it weekly; wash bed sheets and blankets in hot water weekly (temperature of $\geq 130\,°F$ ($55\,°C$) is needed to kill mites) Desirable: • Remove carpets from the bedroom; avoid sleeping or lying on upholstered furniture; remove carpets that are laid on concrete; minimize or wash stuffed toys
Cockroaches	• Use poison bait or traps to control • Do not leave food or garbage exposed • Fix leaky faucets and pipes
Food	• Avoid sulphites and other foods that exacerbate symptoms
Medications	• Counsel patients with severe asthma, nasal polyps, and history of sensitivity to ASA and NSAIDs on severe (and potentially fatal) risks associated with the use of ASA or NSAIDs • Avoid beta-blockers

Asthma Control and Severity

- Complete control (absence of symptoms, no need for rescue medications and normal lung function) is ideal but not achievable in all patients, hence the focus on acceptable control.

- Asthma severity is difficult to assess and may be best determined after asthma is controlled. Once asthma is well controlled, a good way to assess severity is to determine the level of treatment required to sustain acceptable control.

- If control is not adequate, re-assess compliance, inhaler technique, and procedures to eliminate allergens/triggers before modifying treatment.

Table 8. Canadian Criteria for Determining Acceptable Asthma Control
(Boulet 1999; Lemière 2004)

Parameter	Frequency or value
Daytime symptoms	< 4 days/week
Night-time symptoms	< 1 night/week
Physical activity	Normal
Exacerbations	Mild, infrequent
Absent from work or school due to asthma	None
Need for an inhaled short-acting β_2-agonist	< 4 doses/week (may use 1 dose/day to prevent exercise-induced symptoms)
FEV_1 or PEF	≥ 90% of personal best
PEF diurnal variation	< 10-15% (highest PEF − lowest PEF) ÷ highest PEF x 100% for morning and night over a 2-week period

Table 9. Possible Reasons for Poor Asthma Control

Non-compliance, Education, etc.	• Inadequate patient education/perception, especially about "what asthma is, its symptoms, triggers and how it can be controlled" • Patient non-adherence or misunderstanding regarding role and side effects of medications • Poor inhaler technique • Inadequate attention paid to environmental and workplace allergens/triggers (e.g., continued smoking or exposure to smoke, presence of a household pet) • Socioeconomic (e.g., drugs too expensive), psychosocial issues, existing comorbidities • Lack of continuity of care
Additional/Alternate Diagnosis to Asthma and/or Potential Exacerbating Factors	• Some or all of the condition may not be asthma – consider: hyperventilation, GERD, rhinitis, sinusitis, vocal cord dysfunction (see also pages 5, 7 and 8). These conditions may co-exist with asthma, mimic asthma, and potentially make asthma worse • Drugs that exacerbate the condition (e.g., beta-blockers, salicylates, ACE inhibitors)
Inappropriate Asthma Management	• Inappropriate use of corticosteroid agents (e.g., intermittent, no use, or persistent inadequate dose) or lack of add-on therapy (e.g., LABA) • Overuse of β_2-agonists is a sign of poor control
Severe Asthma	• After the above are ruled out, the presence of severe asthma should be considered

Pharmacotherapy of Asthma: Overview [1,2]

(Becker 2005; Boulet 1999; BTS 2005; GINA 2006; Lemière 2004; NAEPP 2002)

Avoidance of asthma allergens/triggers and education should always be emphasized

Inhaled short-acting β_2-agonist (SABA) PRN should always be available for rescue [3]

Therapy	Medications	Asthma Severity
Rescue Therapy	**Inhaled SABA (short-acting β_2-agonist)** As needed for intermittent symptoms and for preventing and treating exercise-induced symptoms [3]	**VERY MILD** (Intermittent symptoms)
Regular Preventer Therapy [4]	**Low-dose ICS (inhaled corticosteroid):** Mainstay of therapy **LTRA (leukotriene receptor antagonist):** Less-effective alternative for those who cannot tolerate or who will not take ICS	**MILD** (Persistent symptoms)
Add-on Therapy	**First-line add-on to ICS: LABA** (long-acting β_2-agonist) • In children [5] usually after moderate doses of ICS (see individual agents for age-specific dosing) • In adults consider after low to moderate doses of ICS • **LABAs should be combined with ICS and never used alone** [6,7] **Second-line add-on to ICS: LTRA** An ICS + LTRA combination is less effective than ICS + LABA **Third-line add-on to ICS: Oral theophylline**	**MODERATE**
Additional Therapy for Persistent Poor Control	**High doses of ICS + LABA** (or ICS + alternative add-on therapies) **Oral prednisone** in very severe cases **Consider anti-IgE therapy** for patients with severe recalcitrant asthma with an allergic component (Table 12)	**SEVERE**

1) Any drug and/or dosage change should be evaluated over a 4-6 week period.

2) Once a patient has achieved and maintained optimal asthma control, attempts should be made to reduce medications within the bounds of acceptable control. Asthma like symptoms spontaneously go into remission in a substantial proportion of children 5 years and younger. Hence the continued need for asthma treatment should be assessed at least twice a year (GINA 2006).

3) The rapid-acting agent Formoterol fumarate dihydrate (Oxeze®), not Formoterol fumarate (Foradil®), may be an alternative. See product monograph for age-specific indications and dosing.

4) Preventer medication (ICS) is suggested when a SABA is used > 3 times/week (aside from 1 pre-exercise dose/day).

5) Children 5 years and younger: No studies on combination therapy, or the addition of LABA, LTRA, or theophylline when patient's asthma not controlled on moderate doses of ICS (GINA 2006).

6) Health Canada Advisory – Safety information about a class of asthma drugs known as long-acting-β_2-agonists. Health Canada. October 4, 2005 (see also SMART trial 2006)

7) ICS/LABA preparations (Advair®, Symbicort®): Check Product Monographs for approved indications and age-specific dosing. A number of studies have been conducted with these combinations with various results including: In moderate to severe persistent asthma, combination ICS/LABA useful when moderate ICS alone is not controlling symptoms. Budesonide/Formoterol in a single inhaler for both maintenance and reliever therapy has demonstrated benefit over fixed-dose combinations plus SABA or Formoterol reliever (O'Byrne 2006; Rabe 2006; Rabe 2006a; Vogelmeier 2005; GINA 2006; Rxfiles.ca).

Table 10. Pharmacotherapy of Asthma: Overview of Acute Rescue Therapy

Short-acting β_2-agonists (SABA)

Medication	Common Dosage Forms and Usual Daily Dosage	Daily Cost
Fenoterol hydrobromide	**pMDI: 100 µg/inhalation** Adults and ≥ 12 years: 1 inhalation as needed. If required, a second inhalation may be taken preferably after waiting 5 minutes. Maximum of 8 inhalations/24 hours	$0.05-0.39
Salbutamol sulfate	**pMDI: 100 µg/inhalation** Adults and Children > 12 years: 1-2 inhalations as needed. To prevent exercise-induced symptoms use 2 inhalations 15-30 minutes prior to exercise. Maximum of 8 inhalations/24 hours	$0.02-0.19
	Children ≥ 4-12 years: 1 inhalation as needed. Increase to 2 inhalations if required. To prevent exercise-induced symptoms use 1 inhalation 15-30 minutes prior to exercise. Increased to 2 inhalations if required. Maximum of 4 inhalations/24 hours	
Terbutaline sulfate	**Turbuhaler® DPI: 500 µg/inhalation** Adults and children ≥ 6 years: 1 inhalation as needed. A second inhalation may be taken preferably after waiting 5 minutes. Maximum of 6 inhalations/24 hours	$0.07-0.43

Table 11. Pharmacotherapy of Asthma: Overview of Regular Preventer Therapy[1, 2, 3, 4, 5]

Inhaled corticosteroids (ICS)

Medication	Common Dosage Forms and Usual Daily Dosage	Daily Cost
Beclomethasone dipropionate	**pMDI: 50 or 100 µg/inhalation** Adults and children ≥ 12 years: 50-400 µg twice daily Children 5-11 years: 50-100 µg twice daily	$0.28-2.27 $0.28-0.57
Budesonide	**Turbuhaler® DPI: 100, 200, or 400 µg/inhalation** Adults and children > 12 years: 200-400 µg twice daily Maximum of 2400 µg/day for severe asthma Children 6-12 years: 100-200 µg twice daily	$0.59-3.19 $0.30-0.59
Ciclesonide	**pMDI: 100 or 200 µg/inhalation** Adults ≥ 18 years: Low to moderate dose: 100-400 µg once daily High dose: 400 µg twice daily	$0.35-1.14 $2.28
Fluticasone propionate	**pMDI: 50, 125, or 250 µg/inhalation** Adults and children > 16 years: 100-500 µg twice daily Children > 4-16 years: 50-100 µg twice daily Children 12 months - 4 years: 50-100 µg twice daily	$0.73-2.40 $0.37-0.73 $0.37-0.73
	Diskus®: 50, 100, 250 or 500 µg/inhalation Adults and children > 16 years: 100-500 µg twice daily Children 4-16 years: 50-200 µg twice daily	$0.99-2.40 $0.55-1.98

1) See Appendix D for trade names and consult latest product monographs for dosing updates. A proposed dose equivalency for ICS is available in Appendix E

2) Inhalation devices are preferred over nebulized solutions (e.g., SABA & ICS). Nebulizers may be considered in patients unable to manipulate an inhaler. See Appendix D for available products and suggested dosing.

3) In younger children (< 5-6 years old), the use of pMDIs with spacers (with or without face mask) is commonly recommended. Typically by 5-6 years children are able to use DPIs (Becker 2005, Dolovich 2005). For further information on inhalation devices refer to the RxFiles (http://www.rxfiles.ca) and/or Canadian Lung Association (http://www.Lung.ca).

4) Although manufacturer recommended doses for adults and children have been included, "auto-scaling" of doses in children may occur. In young children, deposition of medication in the lungs is approximately one-tenth of the dose that would be delivered in adults (Becker 2005). Hence the same dose of maintenance medication may be used for all ages.

5) After maximal improvement is reached, the total daily dose of ICS may be tapered down at a minimum of every two months. The goal of ICS use in asthma management is to achieve control with a low ICS dose. Intermittent therapy is not recommended.

Table 12. Pharmacotherapy of Asthma: Overview of Add-on Therapy [1, 2, 3, 4]

Class	Medication	Common Dosage Forms and Usual Daily Dosage	Daily Cost
Long-acting β_2-agonists (LABA)[5]	Formoterol fumarate dihydrate	**Turbuhaler® DPI: 6 or 12 µg/inhalation** Adults: 6 or 12 µg inhaled every 12 hours Maximum of 48 µg/24 hours	$1.06-1.41
		Children 6-16 yrs: 6 or 12 µg every 12 hours Maximum of 24 µg/24 hours	$1.06-1.41
	Formoterol fumarate	**Aerolizer™: 12 µg capsule for inhalation** Adults and children 6-16 years: 1 capsule inhaled every 12 hours Maximum of 48 µg/24 hours	$1.41-2.82
	Salmeterol xinafoate	**Diskus®, Diskhaler®: 50 µg/inhalation. pMDI: 25 µg/inhalation** Adults and children ≥ 4 years: 50 µg every 12 hours	$1.66
Leukotriene receptor antagonists (LTRA)	Montelukast	Adults and children ≥ 15 years: 10 mg tablet at bedtime	$2.14
		Children 6-14 years: 5 mg chewable tablet at bedtime	$1.45
		Children 2-5 years: 4 mg chewable tablet at bedtime or	$1.32
		4 mg oral granules at bedtime	$1.32
	Zafirlukast	Adults and children ≥ 12 years: 20 mg tablet twice daily	$1.44
Combination Therapy ICS + LABA	Budesonide + Formoterol fumarate dihydrate	**Turbuhaler® DPI: (100 or 200 µg budesonide) + 6 µg formoterol** Adults and children ≥ 12 years: 1 or 2 inhalations (100 or 200 Turbuhaler®) once or twice daily Maximum of 4 inhalations/day	$0.50-2.60
	Fluticasone + Salmeterol xinafoate	**Diskus®: (100, 250, or 500 µg fluticasone) + 50 µg salmeterol** Adults and children ≥ 12 years: 1 inhalation (100, 250, or 500 Diskus®) twice daily	$2.39-4.06
		Children 4-11 years: 1 inhalation (100 Diskus®) twice daily	$2.39
		pMDI: (125 or 250 µg fluticasone) + 25 µg salmeterol Adults and children ≥ 12 years: 2 inhalations (125 or 250 pMDI) twice daily	$1.43-4.06
Xanthine Preparations	Theophylline, Oxtriphylline, Aminophylline	A number of oral products (see Appendix D, F and product monographs for specifics on dosing). Requires monitoring of serum level due to narrow therapeutic index and high potential for drug interactions.	See Appendix D
Corticosteroids	Prednisone	Oral dosage form – use lowest dose possible	
IgE Monoclonal Antibodies (Use needs specialist supervision)	Omalizumab[6]	**Subcutaneous Injection: 150 mg vial** Adults and children ≥ 12 years: Dosing based on body weight and pre-treatment serum IgE concentration. Dosing range from 150 mg subcutaneously every 4 weeks up to a maximum dose of 375 mg subcutaneously every 2 weeks (see product monograph for details).	$21.43-128.57

1) See Appendix D for trade names and consult latest product monographs for dosing updates.

2) In younger children (< 5-6 years old), the use of pMDIs with spacers (with or without face mask) is commonly recommended. Typically by 5-6 years of age children are able use DPIs (Becker 2005, Dolovich 2005). For further information on inhalation devices refer to the RxFiles (http://www.rxfiles.ca) and/or Canadian Lung Association (http://www.lung.ca).

3) Although doses for adults and children have been included, "auto-scaling" of doses in children may occur. In young children, deposition of medication in the lungs is approximately one tenth of the dose that would be delivered in adults (Becker 2005). Hence the same dose of maintenance medication may be used for all ages.

4) **LABAs should be combined with ICS and never used alone (Health Canada 2005; SMART 2006).**

5) The formoterol fumarate dihydrate (Oxeze®) preparation is a long-acting inhaled β_2-agonists (LABA) that exhibits a rapid or fast onset of action and has been referred to as RABA (rapid-acting inhaled β_2-agonist) and FABA (fast-acting inhaled β_2-agonist) (Tattersfield 2001, Astra Product monograph). In asthma patients, ONLY Oxeze® (formoterol fumarate dihydrate) has been approved for rescue therapy and prevention of exercise-symptoms, and not Foradil® (formoterol fumarate). See product monograph for age-specific indications and dosing.

6) Omalizumab is indicated for adults and adolescents (≥ 12 years) with moderate-to-severe persistent asthma who have a positive skin test or in vitro reactivity to a perennial aeroallergen and whose symptoms are inadequately controlled with inhaled corticosteroids. Not to be used for the treatment of acute bronchospasm or status asthmaticus.

Table 13. Pharmacotherapy of Asthma: Other
(Becker 2005; Boulet 1999; Creticos 2000; Lemière 2004)

Category	Indications	Notes
Immunotherapy	Children with established allergic asthma are rarely candidates for immunotherapy and referral to a specialist is suggested.	• The National Asthma Control Task Force recommends that immunotherapy only be administered under the medical supervision of trained personnel in facilities with resuscitative equipment due to potential risks of systemic reactions (e.g., severe and life-threatening systemic anaphylaxis). • Allergen immunotherapy should be combined with allergen avoidance, pharmacotherapy, and patient education. • Immunotherapy is contraindicated in patients with serious cardiovascular comorbidities, uncontrolled hypertension, renal failure, and chronic lung disease (e.g., poorly controlled asthma).

Alternative Therapies

Alternative therapies for asthma exist, but there are few well-controlled studies of such therapies. No objective evidence of benefit was found for these approaches; however, some patients may report a benefit due to a placebo effect. Patients should be made aware that there is a lack of evidence for many of these therapies and reminded not to stop their prescribed asthma medications.

Therapy	Scientific evidence
Acupuncture	No improvement evident in placebo-controlled trials. There may be a small benefit in exercise-induced symptoms.
Buteyko Breathing Techniques	Although Buteyko breathing techniques have not been found to improve measures of lung function, they may play a role in reducing hyperventilation.
Chiropractic	No benefit evident in controlled studies.
Herbal Medicines	No well-controlled, double-blind randomized studies are available.
Homeopathy	A recent double-blind, placebo-controlled trial failed to show any improvement in spirometry or airway hyper-responsiveness. More studies are required.
Hypnosis and Relaxation Techniques	No well controlled, double-blind randomized studies are available. Some open or single-blind studies have suggested a possible role in reducing bronchial hyper-responsiveness.

Acute Exacerbations of Asthma
(Beveridge 1996; Boulet 1999; GINA 2006; NAEPP 1997, 2002)

Exacerbations of asthma (asthma attacks) are considered a **progression of asthma beyond good control of symptoms and/or severe enough to require an increase in medication.**

Patients should be taught:

- How to recognize worsening asthma

- How to treat worsening asthma

- How and when to seek medical attention

In cases of increased severity or exacerbation of symptoms, patients should have **written action plans** for medication self-adjustment, and should document medication requirements for symptom relief.

Severity of exacerbation is assessed through:

- Symptom recognition

- Requirement for frequent SABA

- Decreased response to SABA

- PEF measurement (< 60% personal best or predicted indicates severe exacerbation)

General management of asthma exacerbations in the emergency department:

- Short-acting inhaled β_2-agonist (SABA) for symptomatic relief

- Systemic corticosteroids for moderate to severe exacerbations, or for those who fail to respond to a SABA

- Short-acting inhaled anticholinergics added to SABA in moderate to severe exacerbations

- Oxygen to relieve hypoxemia for moderate to severe exacerbations

- Monitor response to therapy with serial measurements of lung function

For specific treatment information for patients in the emergency department and hospital, please refer to documents from the Canadian Association of Emergency Physicians - http://www.caep.ca (Beveridge 1996; Boulet 1999).

> **An exacerbation that leads to a visit to the emergency department is often an indication of inadequate long-term asthma control or inadequate plans for handling exacerbations**

Table 14. Exacerbations of Asthma: Hospital Discharge Plan and Follow-up[1,2]
(Boulet 1999, 2001)

Consideration for hospital discharge/admission should be based on results of spirometry (percent of previous best, or percent of predicted or absolute value) and assessment of clinical risk factors for relapse.

Usually require admission to hospital	Possible candidates for discharge	Likely candidates for discharge
Patients with a pre-treatment FEV_1 or PEF below 25% of previous best level or the predicted value (i.e., FEV_1 < 1.0L or PEF < 100L/min) Patients with a post-treatment FEV_1 or PEF below 40% of previous best level or the predicted value (i.e., FEV_1 < 1.6L or PEF < 200 L/min)	Patients with a post-treatment FEV_1 or PEF between 40% and 60% of previous best level or predicted value (i.e., FEV_1 = 1.6-2.1 L or PEF = 200-300 L/min)	Patients with a post-treatment FEV_1 or PEF above 60% of previous best level or predicted value (i.e., FEV_1 > 2.1 L or PEF > 300 L/min)

Recommended Discharge Treatment and Follow-up

Treatment	Adults	Children
After discharge, patients should continue systemic glucocorticosteroids (e.g., oral prednisone).	30-60 mg/day for 7-14 days. No tapering required.	1-2 mg/kg/day for 3-5 days. Maximum 50 mg. No tapering required.
Inhaled corticosteroids	Should be prescribed for all patients at discharge or consider increasing the dose of the patient's current inhaled corticosteroid. (including those receiving oral prednisone)	
Follow-up	A treatment plan and clear instructions for follow-up with the family physician is recommended.	

1) **Referral to an asthma education clinic is suggested for ALL patients with high risk factors, poor lung function or indications of chronic poor control.** Risk factors for relapse include: exacerbation requiring an emergency room visit within the past year, recent use of systemic corticosteroids, use of multiple classes of asthma medication, and history of severe or life-threatening asthma attack.

2) Antibiotic therapy is not usually required unless bacterial pneumonia or sinusitis is suspected (e.g., patient presents with fever, purulent discharge, etc.).

Asthma and Pregnancy
(Boulet 1999; Bracken 2003; Luskin 1999; NAEPP 2004; Rey 2007)

Maternal and Fetal Risks	**Poorly controlled asthma during pregnancy can result in serious complications including:** Pre-eclampsia, placenta previa, vaginal hemorrhage, and toxemia. Risks to the fetus include intrauterine growth retardation, reduced birth weight, hypoxia, and perinatal death. Hence, it is imperative to ensure that symptoms are controlled.
Evaluation	**Spirometry, peak flow measurements, and evaluation of symptoms** are considered central in the diagnosis and ongoing assessment of asthma severity. **Fetal oxygenation can be indirectly assessed** using these endpoints.
Asthma Triggers	Assessment and **avoidance of asthma triggers** continues to be an integral component of asthma management. Although successful immunotherapy initiated prior to pregnancy can continue, it is generally not recommended that it be started during this time.
Pharmacotherapy (see Appendix H for further information)	**The approach to pharmacotherapy does not change drastically during pregnancy.** Step-wise increases and decreases in treatment are advocated. Instruct patients to use β_2-agonists as rescue therapy. Inhaled corticosteroids are not contraindicated, and should be prescribed if symptoms warrant. Budesonide has been shown to be safe when used during pregnancy, and should be considered if treatment is to be initiated during pregnancy. Patients do not need to be switched to budesonide if their asthma is well controlled with another ICS. Although causality has not been established, extended use of oral corticosteroids to control severe asthma has been associated with an increased risk of pre-eclampsia, preterm births, hyperbilirubinemia, and perinatal mortality. All patients should be educated that the **minimal risks associated with pharmacotherapy are far outweighed by the risk posed to the mother and infant by uncontrolled asthma.**
Written Action Plan and Follow-up	**A written action plan should be developed with all patients** detailing the management of exacerbations. Inhaled β_2-agonist and courses of corticosteroid therapy continue to be the cornerstone of management, and when necessary oxygen supplementation and prompt emergency care in severe exacerbations. **Regular follow-up throughout the pregnancy should be emphasized, especially if frequent exacerbations or poor control is present.**

CHRONIC OBSTRUCTIVE PULMONARY DISEASE (COPD)

OVERVIEW - General Characteristics of COPD

Age of Onset	• Usually in patients between 35 to 40 years of age (onset in women may be younger than men) • Screening for α_1-antitrypsin deficiency is recommended for patients with atypical features of COPD, including patients with early-onset disease, a positive family history, or those who become disabled in their 40s or 50s. However, α_1-antitrypsin deficiency accounts for only 1 to 2% of COPD
Role of Smoking to Disease	• Directly related, usually > 10 pack-years • The most important causative agent in 80-90% of all COPD cases in North America • Other factors include occupation, air pollution, and/or exposure to biomass fuels used for cooking and heating in poorly ventilated dwellings
History of Allergy	• Unrelated, may or may not be present
Family History	• Occasionally • α_1-antitrypsin deficiency is inherited • Genetics of COPD being studied
Symptoms	• Dyspnea and activity limitation
Disease Course	• Slow, cumulative, progressive and associated with frequent exacerbations
Spirometry	• Key element in diagnosis and monitoring disease progression • Minimal changes in spirometry with effective therapy
Reversibility of Airflow Obstruction	• Airflow obstruction is chronic, progressive and persistent, but partially reversible even in advanced disease. FEV_1 always reduced if disease significant • FEV_1 generally poorly responsive, but may improve with bronchodilators in some patients • Symptom response, including exercise capacity, rather than FEV_1 responsiveness, is the best way to assess the value of bronchodilator therapy
Hypoxemia	• Chronic in advanced stages (in minority)
Chest X-ray	• Often normal in early disease • When abnormality present, increased bronchial markings (chronic bronchitis) and chronic hyperinflation (emphysema) often co-exist • Not diagnostic; useful to rule out other diseases

OVERVIEW - Management of COPD

Prevention	• Smoking cessation • Immunization (prevent exacerbations)
Non-pharmacological Therapy	• Pulmonary rehabilitation • Education • Nutrition • Psychosocial support
Pharmacotherapy (Treatment options for reaching acceptable symptom control)	1) SABA prn and/or regularly scheduled short acting anticholinergic 2) (Long-acting inhaled anticholinergic or LABA) plus SABA prn 3) (Long-acting inhaled anticholinergic and LABA) plus SABA prn 4) Consider adding ICS in those with moderate to severe COPD with 1 or more exacerbations per year 5) Long-acting oral theophylline may be considered in severe disease when dyspnea persists despite maximal combined inhaler therapy
Response to Therapy as Measured by Spirometry and Symptoms	• Minimal changes in spirometry with effective therapy • Goal is symptom improvement and increased functional capacity
Adjunctive Therapy	• Oxygen supplementation • If necessary, surgical therapies: Lung volume reduction surgery, bullectomy, lung transplantation
Acute Exacerbations	• Bronchodilators • Antibiotic treatment of bacterial infections – purulent exacerbations • Systemic corticosteroids if moderate or more severe (e.g., $FEV_1 < 60\%$ predicted) • Oxygen supplementation as needed

Legend	
Anticholinergics	Short-acting (ipratropium); Long-acting (tiotropium)
ICS	Inhaled Corticosteroid (e.g., beclomethasone, budesonide, fluticasone)
LABA	Long-acting Inhaled β_2-agonists (e.g., formoterol, salmeterol)
SABA	Short-acting Inhaled β_2-agonists (e.g., fenoterol, salbutamol, terbutaline)

Background

Definition

COPD refers to "a respiratory disorder largely caused by smoking, which is characterized by progressive, partially reversible airway obstruction, systemic manifestations, and increasing frequency and severity of exacerbations". Although COPD is predominantly caused by smoking, other factors (environmental/occupational) may contribute to its development.

Many physicians are familiar with COPD being categorized as "chronic bronchitis" or "emphysema". Chronic bronchitis and emphysema both occur in COPD; however, both may be present in the absence of airflow obstruction and the diagnosis of COPD. These terms should NOT BE USED to define and manage COPD (O'Donnell 2003, 2004).

Mortality/Morbidity

In Canada, chronic obstructive pulmonary disease (COPD) accounted for 4% (n = 9041) of all deaths in 1998. This may be an underestimate of the actual mortality rate, because although COPD may be listed on the death certificate as the "underlying cause of death", the "primary cause of death" may be listed as another condition (e.g., pneumonia or congestive heart failure). COPD plays a significant role in overall deaths between the ages of 65 and 84 (CIHI 2001). From 1998 to 1999, mortality rates in women increased by 53% compared to a 7% decrease in men. The morbidity and mortality from COPD is predicted to increase over the next 15 years, especially in aging females (O'Donnell 2003, 2004). Estimates from existing data indicate that more women are losing their lives to COPD than to breast cancer (CIHI 2001, CCS/NCIC 2006).

Prevalence

According to the 1998/99 National Population Health Survey (NPHS), 3.2% of Canadians 35 years or older (211,900 men and 286,600 women) had chronic bronchitis or emphysema diagnosed by a health professional, a number that is likely an underestimate of the true prevalence of COPD. **It is estimated that at least 50% of patients who have COPD remain undiagnosed.** COPD is currently the fourth most common cause of death in the world and is expected to continue rising in prevalence to become the third most common cause of death in the next 10 to 15 years. The demographics are changing dramatically so that in Canada, more women than men suffer from the disease are more likely to be hospitalized for its care. Because women are more susceptible to the adverse effects of tobacco smoke than men, their disease manifests at an earlier age, often while women are active in the workforce (CIHI 2001).

Health Care Services and Costs

In 1997 the average in-hospital length of stay due to COPD in Canada was reported as 10.5 days. The economic burden of COPD reported in 1998 was estimated at $1.67 billion and included drug and hospital care expenditures and indirect costs. The true costs are probably higher, as this figure does not take into account the cost of physicians or costs related to community-based health services.

PART I
Diagnosis of COPD

Diagnosis of COPD (O'Donnell 2003, 2004)

- The key symptoms seen with COPD are **shortness of breath and activity limitation.** The symptoms **usually manifest slowly and are cumulative, progressive and associated with frequent exacerbations.**

- At first COPD is confined to the lungs but in advanced stages COPD can be accompanied by altered nutritional status, depression, right heart failure, secondary polycythemia, and skeletal muscle dysfunction.

- Advanced COPD is associated with multiple comorbidities (i.e., cardiovascular disease, osteoporosis, thromboembolic disease, diabetes, and lung cancer).

- The diagnosis of COPD **requires** spirometry to objectively demonstrate airflow obstruction. Two measurements are necessary to establish the diagnosis of COPD (See Table 1 and 2).

> **Family Practitioners have an important role in the early diagnosis and management of COPD. Many COPD patients are not diagnosed until the disease is well advanced. Hence targeted spirometry for individuals at risk is paramount (O'Donnell 2003, 2004).**

Table 1. Clinical Assessment
(O'Donnell 2003, 2004)

1) History

☐ Quantify tobacco consumption

$$\text{Total pack years} = \frac{\text{\# of cigarettes smoked / day}}{20\,*} \times \text{\# years of smoking}$$

* although the number of cigarettes per pack may vary between different countries (e.g., 20, 25) the above standardized equation uses 20 per pack to maintain consistency

☐ Assess **severity of dyspnea and disability** (see page 29 for MRC scale)

☐ Assess **frequency and severity of exacerbations** (may help guide treatment)

☐ Note any **occupational / environmental exposures** to lung irritants

☐ Presence of **other chronic lung diseases, family history of COPD**

☐ Co-morbidities (anxiety, depression, cardiovascular disease, osteoporosis, thromboembolic disease, diabetes, lung cancer)

2) Physical Exam

☐ Important, however, usually not diagnostic and can underestimate presence of significant airflow limitation

☐ In advanced disease may note signs of lung hyperinflation, right heart failure, and generalized muscle wasting

3) Investigations

☐ **Spirometry** – FEV_1 and FEV_1 / FVC are the best measures (see Table 2)

☐ **Chest X-rays** – not diagnostic but useful to rule out co-morbidities

☐ **Arterial blood gas measurements** should be offered to patients with $FEV_1 < 40\%$ predicted or when respiratory failure is suspected

☐ **Screening for α_1-antitrypsin deficiency** is recommended for patients with atypical features of COPD, including patients with early-onset disease, a positive family history, or those who become disabled in their 40s or 50s. A blood test is required for screening. Contact your local laboratory for details.

Table 2. Spirometry
(O'Donnell 2003, 2004)

Mass screening of asymptomatic individuals for COPD is not supported by the current evidence and is therefore not recommended.

- **Suspect COPD and perform spirometry in:**
  - Current or past smokers* who are 35** years or older
  - Individuals with persistent cough and sputum production
  - Individuals who experience frequent and/or persistent respiratory tract infections
  - Individuals with progressive activity-related shortness of breath
  - Individuals who have significant occupational exposure to respiratory irritants
  - Individuals thought initially to have asthma but responding sub-optimally to therapy

    * Second-hand smoke may also have an impact, but the extent of this is currently not well known

    ** (NZ/Australia: 35 years) (O'Donnell et al, 2003, 2004: 40 years)

- **Spirometry is necessary** (includes measurement of FEV_1 and FVC) to establish the diagnosis of COPD as well as in the assessment of severity, progression and prognosis.

- **Airflow obstruction is defined as a post bronchodilator FEV_1 < 80 % of the predicted value in association with an FEV_1/FVC ratio < 0.7. <u>BOTH are necessary to establish a diagnosis of COPD.</u>**

- Due to possible fluctuation in airflow obstruction measures (FEV_1 and FVC) **it is possible that the diagnosis of COPD cannot be established after the first evaluation** and subsequent spirometry may be required.

- **Spirometric assessment can be undertaken at a family practice site, in a specialist center or hospital.** The accuracy depends on proper training, adequate application of good technique, calibration, and maintenance of equipment. For further information on spirometry see Appendix A.

- **Full pulmonary function testing (PFT) with measurement of diffusion capacity and lung volumes is <u>NOT usually required in the family practice setting</u>** (full PFTs are recommended if dyspnea intensity appears disproportionately increased while spirometry is relatively preserved).

FEV_1 = Forced expiratory volume in 1 second   FVC = Forced Vital Capacity

Table 3. Differential Diagnosis of COPD/Chronic Breathlessness
(O'Donnell 2004)

- A number of other conditions can be included in the differential diagnosis of COPD/chronic breathlessness including: anemia, asthma, bronchiectasis, bronchiolitis obliterans, congestive heart failure, cystic fibrosis, obesity, pulmonary vascular disease (emboli), and tuberculosis.
- It is important to differentiate between asthma and COPD as the treatment and prognosis are different. Noted below are key differences:

	Asthma	COPD
Age of Onset	• Any age, usually < 40 years • Symptoms often first appear in childhood	• Usually appears between 35 to 40 years (onset in women may younger than men) • In those diagnosed under age 45 years, suspect α_1-antitrypsin deficiency – even earlier if the patient also smokes. However most patients do not have α_1-antitrypsin deficiency
Role of Smoking	• Not directly related but accelerates decline in lung function • Smoking adversely affects the condition and response to therapy • Maternal smoking increases the likelihood of wheezing in childhood • Consider second-hand smoke	• Directly related, usually > 10 pack-years • The most important causative agent in 80-90% of all COPD cases in North America • Other factors include occupation, air pollution, or exposure to biomass fuels used for cooking and heating in poorly ventilated dwellings
History of Allergy	• More likely • Aspirin sensitivity triad: nasal polyps, rhinitis, ASA intolerance	• Unrelated, may or may not be present
Family History	• Yes, a risk factor for asthma is parental history of asthma or eczema	• Occasionally • α_1-antitrypsin deficiency is inherited
Symptoms	• Wheezing, chest tightness, dyspnea, cough, and infrequent sputum production • Intermittent, variable, often paroxysmal and provoked by allergic or non-allergic stimuli (e.g., cold air, irritants, viruses) • Frequently nocturnal • Exercise-induced bronchoconstriction may occur	• Dyspnea and activity limitation
Disease Course	• Usually stable with exacerbations	• Slow, cumulative, progressive and associated with frequent exacerbations
Spirometry	• Key element in diagnosis (in older asthmatics) and to confirm an adequate response to therapy	• Key element in diagnosis and monitoring disease progression
Reversibility of Airflow Obstruction	• Airflow obstruction is usually episodic and completely reversible with therapy • FEV_1 usually normal between attacks or quickly improves with bronchodilators • Normal FEV_1 may not be achievable in long-standing asthma, especially if poorly controlled	• Airflow obstruction is chronic, progressive, and persistent, but partially reversible even in advanced disease. FEV_1 always reduced if disease significant • FEV_1 generally poorly responsive, but may improve with bronchodilators in some patients • Symptom response, including exercise capacity, rather than FEV_1 responsiveness is the best way to assess the value of bronchodilator therapy
Hypoxemia	• Unusual; episodic with severe attacks	• Chronic in advanced stages (in minority)
Chest X-ray	• Usually normal except during acute attacks	• Often normal in early disease • When abnormality present, increased bronchial markings (chronic bronchitis) and chronic hyperinflation (emphysema) often co-exist • Not diagnostic – useful to rule out other diseases

Stratifying/Classifying Severity in COPD

- **Classification and management of COPD is largely driven by symptoms.** The Medical Research Council (MRC) Dyspnea scale (Figure 1) can be used to assess shortness of breath and disability, help identify patients with poor quality of life and provide prognostic information on survival.

- Classification of COPD severity in patients with co-morbid disease (e.g., cardiac, anemia, metabolic disorders, muscle weakness) is difficult and should be undertaken with care as symptoms may not appropriately reflect COPD severity.

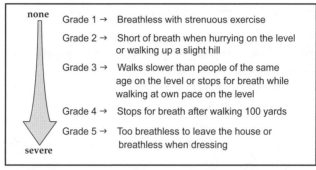

| none |
| severe |

Grade 1 →	Breathless with strenuous exercise
Grade 2 →	Short of breath when hurrying on the level or walking up a slight hill
Grade 3 →	Walks slower than people of the same age on the level or stops for breath while walking at own pace on the level
Grade 4 →	Stops for breath after walking 100 yards
Grade 5 →	Too breathless to leave the house or breathless when dressing

Figure 1. The Medical Research Council (MRC) dyspnea scale is used to assess shortness of breath and disability in chronic obstructive pulmonary disease (O'Donnell 2003, 2004, originally Fletcher 1959).

Table 4. COPD Classification by Symptoms / Disability
(O'Donnell 2003, 2004; Chapman 2006)

COPD Stage	Common Symptoms
At Risk (does not fulfill the criteria for diagnosis of COPD)	• At risk individuals can include: asymptomatic smokers, ex-smokers; those with chronic productive cough, dyspnea; those who have exposure to pollutants and/or have a family history of respiratory disease • $FEV_1 \geq 80\%$ and/or $FEV_1/FVC \geq 0.7$
Mild (MRC 2)	• Shortness of breath when walking quickly, climbing stairs or slight hill
Moderate (MRC 3 & 4)	• Shortness of breath causes patient to stop after walking approximately 100 metres (or after a few minutes) on level ground
Severe (MRC 5)	• Shortness of breath when dressing and too breathless to leave house • Or the presence of chronic respiratory failure or clinical signs of right heart failure (non-MRC criteria)

Table 5. COPD Classification of Severity of Airflow Obstruction
(O'Donnell 2003, 2004)

Airflow Obstruction	Post-bronchodilator Spirometry
Mild	$FEV_1 = 60\text{-}79\%$ predicted and $FEV_1/FVC < 0.7$
Moderate	$FEV_1 = 40\text{-}59\%$ predicted and $FEV_1/FVC < 0.7$
Severe	$FEV_1 < 40\%$ predicted and $FEV_1/FVC < 0.7$

- **There is a poor relationship between symptoms and degree of airflow limitation.**
- Different spirometric thresholds for severity of disease have been recommended, but have not been clinically validated. **FEV_1 measurement may correlate poorly with symptom severity, exercise capacity and quality of life.** However, it remains necessary for diagnostic and follow-up purposes.

When to Consider Referral to a Specialist
(ATS 2005; CTS 2003)

- **Diagnosis is uncertain or challenging** (e.g, those with chronic asthma who are smokers)
- **Symptoms are severe or inconsistent** with the severity of the air flow obstruction on spirometry
- In the presence of **accelerated decline in lung function (FEV$_1$) of $\geq$ 80 mL per year over a two year period**
- Onset of symptoms occurring at a **young age** (< 35 years)
- **Specialist can also assist where:**
  - COPD patient fails to respond to combined bronchodilator therapy
  - Severe or recurrent exacerbations occur
  - COPD patient has complex comorbidities
  - Pulmonary rehabilitation is required
  - Assessment for oxygen is required
  - Surgical therapies (lung volume reduction surgery, bullectomy, lung transplantation) are a possibility
  - α_1-antitrypsin deficiency is present

PART II
Management of COPD

COPD Management: Goals and Objectives

COPD is characterized by airflow obstruction and by definition is a chronic and progressive disorder, but remains partially reversible even in advanced disease. **Complete resolution** of the patient's symptoms and reversal of damage **is not a realistic goal of treatment.** However, it is usually possible to significantly improve dyspnea and exertional endurance and thus improve quality of life for these patients.

The overall goal is to improve health status and the quality of life of COPD patients, as well as to reduce hospitalizations, morbidity, and early mortality. A practical approach to manage the disease is described below:

1. Prevent further lung damage

- Smoking cessation
- Avoidance of occupational and air pollutants (includes second-hand smoke)
- Immunization
- Preventing and treating exacerbations

2. Optimize current lung function and improve symptoms

- Education
- Pulmonary rehabilitation
- Pharmacological therapy
- Oxygen supplementation
- Surgical approaches (lung volume reduction surgery, bullectomy, lung transplantation)

COPD

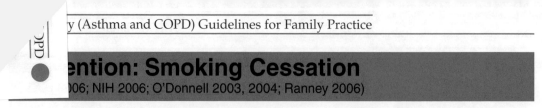

ention: Smoking Cessation
006; NIH 2006; O'Donnell 2003, 2004; Ranney 2006)

Smoking is considered the single most important cause of COPD with 80-90% of all COPD cases in North America being attributable to tobacco exposure. Smoking cessation is the most effective intervention for reducing the risk of developing COPD and for slowing down its progression.

- The greater the exposure, the greater the risk of developing airway obstruction (Figure 2).

- One-half of smokers develop chronic bronchitis and approximately 15-20% develop chronic airflow obstruction.

- After quitting smoking, the rate of decline in FEV_1 returns towards that of a nonsmoker (Figure 3), thus helping to avoid early disability and death due to lung disease. Quitting smoking should also produce symptomatic relief of chronic cough, sputum expectoration, shortness of breath, and wheezing.

- In older patients with well-established or advanced disease, airway inflammation persists despite smoking cessation. However, stopping smoking at the later stages of COPD reduces the risks of developing cardiovascular disease and cancer.

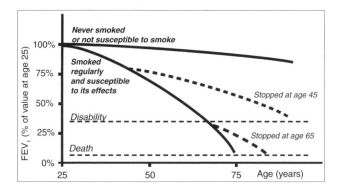

Figure 2. Effects of Smoking Smoking Cessation on Rate of Decline of FEV_1
(O'Donnell 2003, 2004; originally Fletcher 1977)

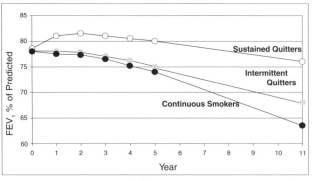

Figure 3. Average Post-Bronchodilator FEV_1
Values expressed as a percentage of predicted normal are values shown over 11 years of study among continuing smokers, intermittent quitters and sustained quitters. (O'Donnell 2003, 2004; originally Anthonisen 2002)

Prevention: Smoking Cessation Strategies

Smoking cessation is not an easy task for patients. On an annual basis, nearly one-half of smokers attempt to quit, but only 7% are still abstinent a year later.

Unplanned attempts: Two recent reports (Larabie 2005; West 2006) found that unplanned attempts to quit smoking were common (approximately one-half of attempts involved no previous planning). An unplanned quit attempt has been defined as a sudden decision not to smoke any more cigarettes, and may be triggered by some unforeseen event (e.g., myocardial infarction). Unplanned (vs. planned) quit attempts were reported as more likely to succeed for at least 6 months (West 2006).

Planned attempts: Changes in behaviour in planned attempts of smoking cessation have been classically described using Prochaska's "Stages of change" model.

Table 6. Prochaska's "Stages of Change" Model Regarding Smoking Cessation
(O'Donnell 2004)

1. **Precontemplation** (not considering stopping in next 6 months)
   - Help the smoker start thinking about quitting
2. **Contemplation** (thinking about stopping within 6 months)
   - Assist the smoker in making the decision to stop
3. **Preparation** (having decided to stop within the next month)
   - Assist in setting a target date for quitting and discuss concerns
4. **Action** (having stopped)
   - Smoker who has stopped should be congratulated and continually supported
5. **Maintenance** (not having smoked for 6 months or more)
   - Review the reasons to quit, discuss actual and future benefits; encourage lifestyle change

---

The Tobacco Use and Dependence Clinical Practice Guideline Panel, Staff, and Consortium Representatives of the U.S. Public Health Service published the "5 As", strategies for helping a willing patient cease tobacco use (GOLD 2006; U.S. Public Service 2000).

Table 7. Strategies for Helping a Willing Patient Cease Tobacco Use – the "5 As"

1. **ASK – Systematically identify all tobacco users at every office visit**
2. **ADVISE – Strongly urge all tobacco users to quit**
3. **ASSESS – Determine the patient's willingness to try to quit**
4. **ASSIST – Help the patient with a quitting plan**
5. **ARRANGE – Schedule follow-up**

Prevention: Smoking Cessation Strategies

Table 8. Factors that Increase Smoking Cessation Rates
(Hughes 2004; O'Donnell 2004; Silagy 2004; van der Meer 2000)

- Consistent advice and reinforcement from physicians (stronger evidence) and other health professionals.

- Individual and group counselling sessions.

- Longer session times (> 10 minutes was best); however, even a brief 3 minute counselling session that urges a smoker to quit can be effective, and should be included at each visit and patients reminded that more intensive therapy increases the likelihood of sustained quitting.

- Longer total person-to-person contact time (31-90 minutes).

- Greater number of sessions (> 8 sessions was best).

- Discussing high-risk situations, developing coping skills and anticipating relapse. Encourage patients to be persistent despite failures, as long-term cessation typically takes 3 to 4 attempts.

- Avoid 'cutting back' strategy. In the short term, smokers who reduce the number of cigarettes they smoke will unconsciously adjust their smoking pattern to maintain their nicotine levels (i.e., deeper puffs, longer breath-holds). In the long term, smokers who reduce their consumption eventually return to their usual level of consumption.

- Initiating pharmacotherapy when counselling is not sufficient (e.g., nicotine replacement therapy, bupropion, nortriptyline or varenicline*). Special consideration should be given before using pharmacotherapy in people smoking fewer than 10 cigarettes per day, pregnant women, adolescents, and those with medical contraindications (e.g., nicotine replacement is contraindicated in patients with unstable angina, untreated peptic ulcer, recent MI/stroke and severe cardiac arrhythmia and bupropion is contraindicated in patients with history of seizures).

*For further details on pharmacotherapy in smoking cessation see http://www.RxFiles.com.

For further information on Smoking Cessation Strategies see a recent Systematic Review (Ranney 2006) and NIH Statement 2006. Overall, the systematic review concluded that self-help strategies alone minimally affect quit rates and that combined pharmacotherapies and counseling either alone or in combination can significantly increase cessation rates.

Prevention: Immunization

Influenza vaccination

COPD patients are considered to be in the high-risk group for influenza-related complications (Canadian Immunization Guide 2002). Influenza vaccination decreases serious illness and death in COPD patients by 50% and reduces the incidence of hospitalization by nearly 40% in patients with chronic respiratory illness (GOLD 2006; O'Donnell 2004). **Annual influenza vaccination is recommended for all COPD patients who have no contraindications** (O'Donnell 2004).

Pneumococcal vaccination

The beneficial effects of pneumococcal vaccination in COPD patients are less well established than with influenza vaccination (O'Donnell 2004). Isolation of new strains of *S. pneumoniae* in COPD patients has been associated with acute exacerbations (Sethi 2002) and colonization with *S. pneumoniae* in COPD patients may increase the risk of an exacerbation (Bogaert 2004). Recent evidence suggests that pneumococcal vaccination is effective in select groups of COPD patients < 65 years with severe airflow obstruction (Alfageme 2006). **Overall, pneumococcal vaccination is recommended for all COPD patients who have no contraindications. It should be given at least once in their lives and repeat vaccination be considered in 5 to 10 years for high-risk patients** (O'Donnell 2004).

Table 9. Recommended Vaccinations in COPD Patients			
Vaccine[1]	Dosage	Common Adverse Effects	Contraindications
Influenza	1 dose 0.5 mL IM/SC annually in fall	Fever, chills, malaise, local swelling and/or soreness	• History of anaphylactic reaction or hypersensitivity to eggs or egg products • Sensitivity to thimerosal • Acute febrile illness
Pneumococcal (Pneumovax)	1 dose 0.5 mL IM/SC Consider revaccination every 5-10 years	Local soreness and erythema	• Hypersensitivity to any component of the vaccine or to diphtheria toxoid

1) Vaccines may be given at the same time at different sites and with different syringes, e.g., both arms, with no increase in adverse reactions.

Pulmonary Rehabilitation in COPD
(ATS 2006; O'Donnell 2003, 2004)

A recent statement (ATS 2006) concluded that evidence for improvement in exercise endurance, dyspnea, functional capacity and quality of life is stronger for rehabilitation than for almost any other therapy in COPD, and documentation of its favourable effect on health care utilization is increasing.

It is important to recognize that pulmonary rehabilitation is as valuable as pharmacological approaches when attempting to improve dyspnea, quality of life and exercise tolerance. Hence, a strategy incorporating both non-pharmacological and pharmacological approaches is more likely to improve COPD (O'Donnell 2004).

Patients with advanced COPD are often elderly and may have comorbid illnesses that contribute to their symptoms of disabling dyspnea and poor exertional endurance. They thus have a strong tendency to drift into quite sedentary lifestyles, which can lead to further general and cardiovascular deconditioning, worsening symptoms, and a diminished quality of life.

When properly initiated, a multi-disciplinary approach to pulmonary rehabilitation can enhance the life quality of patients with advanced COPD despite no measurable improvement in lung function parameters.

However, access to a formal pulmonary rehabilitation program is not always possible or necessary to achieve gratifying gains in activities of daily living. Simpler forms of this type of non-drug oriented therapy using a self-directed approach may be effective in selected cases.

To prevent a return to a sedentary lifestyle and loss of the physical conditioning gains, the following are recommended:

- Constant encouragement and reassurance from the physician for both the patient and the caregiver

- Simple walking and/or stair climbing regimens

- Community resources which can help organize and encourage such self-directed programs include the local Lung Association and physiotherapy groups and many geriatric programs

In addition, by optimizing the pharmacological management of COPD, it is often possible to reduce symptoms sufficiently to permit patients to increase their levels of activity gradually.

Education / Nutrition / Rehabilitation Programs
(Bourbeau 2003, 2004; O'Donnell 2003, 2004)

1. Education and Self-Management Plans

- **Education of the patient and family** with supervision and support based on disease-specific self-management principles is invaluable. These programs can produce a marked reduction in the use of health care services and costs.

- **A comprehensive self management plan** has been shown to improve quality of life, emergency visits, unscheduled physician visits, and hospitalization for COPD exacerbations.

2. Nutritional Therapy and Counselling

- **Consider functional and nutritional status during assessment**, especially in elderly or isolated persons.

- **Malnutrition is an independent risk factor for poor prognosis**, independent of FEV_1.

- **Both obesity and loss of body mass are associated with poor prognosis in COPD**, independent of FEV_1. Undernourished patients commonly suffer respiratory muscle dysfunction and increased mortality.

- **Nutritional counselling, appropriate weight loss or nutritional supplementation can significantly improve symptoms of COPD.**

3. Physical Rehabilitation / Exercise Training

- **Lower extremity training:** This includes walking, cycle ergometry, and treadmill walking and has been shown to significantly improve quality of life, peak exercise capacity, walking distance, and endurance times. There was also a trend towards reduced mortality, decreased hospital days, fewer exacerbations and more efficient primary care use.

- **Upper extremity training and strength training:** Though both are suggested in rehabilitation programs their impact beyond the effect of lower extremity training is not clear.

- **Encouragement to resume regular physical activities as soon as possible after exacerbations.**

Pharmacotherapy of Stable COPD - Overview

Encourage smoking cessation, vaccination, and pulmonary rehabilitation.

Short-acting inhaled β₂-agonist (SABA) PRN always available as rescue medication.

Increasing Severity of Symptoms →

Severity of Symptoms	Management
MILD (with activity-related breathlessness and minimal disability)	**SABA PRN** and/or **Short-acting inhaled anticholinergic**
MILD (if symptoms persist)	CHANGE TO: **Long-acting inhaled anticholinergic** or **Long-acting Inhaled β₂-agonist (LABA)** *Long-acting preparations should not replace SABAs for rescue*
MODERATE (persistent symptoms and exercise intolerance)	COMBINE **Long-acting inhaled anticholinergic** and **LABA**
MODERATE TO SEVERE COPD WITH ≥ 1 EXACERBATIONS PER YEAR (especially where exacerbations required oral corticosteroids)	ADD **Inhaled corticosteroids (ICS)** (Consider combination products for convenience for those already receiving these medications separately)
SEVERE (when dyspnea persists despite maximal combined inhaler therapy)	ADD TRIAL OF **Long-acting oral theophylline**

- If one bronchodilator fails, ensure that the patient is compliant and able to use the prescribed delivery system properly.
- If a medication does not improve the patient's symptoms despite proper use, consider discontinuing the medication.
- Patients may be able to perceive that their symptoms are worse when a medication is discontinued, more than they can attribute a benefit from a medication.

Table 10. Pharmacotherapy of Stable COPD: Overview of Agents [1,2]

Class	Medication	Common Dosage Forms and Usual Daily Dosage	Daily Cost
Short-acting β_2-agonists (SABA)	Fenoterol hydrobromide	**pMDI: 100 µg/inhalation** 1 inhalation as needed. If required, a second inhalation may be taken preferably after waiting 5 minutes. Maximum of 8 inhalations/24 hours	$0.15-0.39
	Salbutamol sulfate	**pMDI: 100 µg/inhalation** 1-2 inhalations as needed. To prevent exercise-induced symptoms use 2 inhalations 15-30 minutes prior to exercise. Maximum of 8 inhalations/24 hours	$0.09-0.19
	Terbutaline sulfate	**Turbuhaler® DPI: 0.5 mg/inhalation** 1 inhalation as needed. A second inhalation may be taken preferably after waiting 5 minutes. Maximum of 6 inhalations/24 hours	$0.07-0.43
Short-acting Inhaled Anticholinergic	Ipratropium bromide	**pMDI: 20 µg/inhalation** 2-4 inhalations 3-4 times/day Maximum of 12 inhalations/24 hours	$0.47-0.95
Long-acting Inhaled Anticholinergic	Tiotropium bromide monohydrate	**HandiHaler®: 18 µg capsule for inhalation** 1 capsule inhaled daily	$2.10

1) See Appendix D for trade names and consult latest product monographs for dosing updates.

2) Inhalation devices are preferred over nebulized solutions (e.g., SABA & ICS). Nebulizers may be considered in patients unable to manipulate an inhaler. See Appendix D for available products. For information on inhalation devices refer to the RxFiles (http://www.rxfiles.ca) and/or Canadian Lung Association (http://www.lung.ca).

Table 11. Pharmacotherapy of Stable COPD: Overview of Agents [1,2]

Class	Medication	Common Dosage Forms and Usual Daily Dosage	Daily Cost
Long-acting Inhaled β_2-agonists (LABA)	Formoterol fumarate dihydrate	**Turbuhaler® DPI: 6 or 12 µg/inhalation** 6 or 12 µg inhaled every 12 hours Maximum of 48 µg/24 hours	$1.06-2.82
	Formoterol fumarate	**Aerolizer™:12 µg capsule for inhalation** 1 or 2 capsules inhaled every 12 hours Maximum of 48 µg/24 hours	$1.41-2.82
	Salmeterol xinafoate	**Diskus®, Diskhaler®: 50 µg/inhalation** **pMDI: 25 µg/inhalation** 50 µg every 12 hours	$1.66
Inhaled Corticosteroids (ICS)	Beclomethasone dipropionate	**pMDI: 50 or 100 µg/inhalation** 50-400 µg twice daily Maximum of 800 µg/24 hours	$0.28-2.27
	Budesonide	**Turbuhaler® DPI: 100, 200, or 400 µg/inhalation** 200-400 µg twice daily Maximum of 2400 µg/24 hours	$0.59-3.19
	Fluticasone propionate	**pMDI: 50, 125, or 250 µg/inhalation** 100-500 µg twice daily Maximum of 1000 µg/24 hours	$0.73-2.40
		Diskus®: 50, 100, 250 or 500 µg/inhalation 100-500 µg twice daily Maximum of 1000 µg/24 hours	$0.99-2.40
Combination Therapy ICS + LABA	Budesonide + Formoterol fumarate dihydrate	**Turbuhaler® DPI: 200 µg budesonide + 6 µg formoterol [3]** 2 inhalations twice daily Maximum of 4 inhalations/day	$2.60
	Fluticasone + Salmeterol xinafoate	**Diskus®: (250 or 500 µg fluticasone) + 50 µg salmeterol** 1 inhalation (250 or 500 Diskus®) twice daily	$2.86-4.06
Xanthine Preparations	Theophylline, Oxtriphylline, Aminophylline	A number of oral products (see Appendix D, F and product monographs for specifics on dosing). Requires monitoring of serum level due to narrow therapeutic index and high potential for drug interactions.	See Appendix D

1) See Appendix D for trade names and consult latest product monographs for dosing updates.

2) Inhalation devices are preferred over nebulized solutions (e.g. SABA & ICS). Nebulizers may be considered in patients unable to manipulate an inhaler. See Appendix D for available products. For information on inhalation devices refer to the RxFiles (http://www.rxfiles.ca) and/or Canadian Lung Association (http:/www.lung.ca).

3) Dosage as used in published clinical trials (Calverley 2003; Szafranski 2003).

Role of Corticosteroids in COPD

Oral Corticosteroids

Long-term use of oral corticosteroids is currently not recommended in COPD patients.

- Long-term use of oral corticosteroids often causes unacceptable side effects (e.g., weight gain, hypertension, osteoporosis, cataracts, immunosuppression, thin skin, avascular necrosis of the hip). Long-term use does not appear to prevent worsening of COPD (Walters 2005).

- A short course of high dose oral corticosteroids can reduce the duration of acute exacerbations. Consider adding systemic corticosteroids (prednisone 25-50 mg daily x 7-14 days); they are of benefit in moderate to severe exacerbations (i.e., $FEV_1 < 50\%$ predicted in outpatients and AECOPD that require hospitalization) (Aaron 2003; Davies 1999; O'Donnell 2003).

Inhaled Corticosteroids

Inhaled corticosteroids should be considered for patients with more advanced COPD who have ONE or more exacerbations per year, and should be given in combination with long-acting bronchodilators. There is no evidence for their use as monotherapy in patients with COPD.

- Regular treatment with inhaled corticosteroids has not been shown to slow the decline in lung function or reliably improve the quality of life (O'Donnell 2004).

- In the large subgroup of patients who did not improve significantly with an oral corticosteroid, inhaled corticosteroids, even at high doses, failed to show beneficial physiological and functional effects in those with advanced COPD already on bronchodilator therapy (Bourbeau 1998).

- In the few studies where patients with COPD were selected according to a significant spirometric response to oral corticosteroids, less than 50% of study participants using inhaled corticosteroids were able to achieve or to maintain at least 50% of the improvement in spirometry that they had on oral corticosteroids (Shim 1985; Bourbeau 1993).

- If the patient is normally treated with an inhaled corticosteroid, it would seem reasonable to maintain the patient on both oral and inhaled corticosteroids during acute exacerbations. Inhaled steroids have no role in treating exacerbations, but when used regularly may reduce the frequency of exacerbations in patients with more severe COPD (i.e., with frequent exacerbations, poor lung function = $FEV_1 < 50\%$ predicted) (Burge 2000/ISOLDE).

- Please refer to Appendix G for safety issues regarding corticosteroids.

Acute Exacerbations of Chronic Bronchitis (AECB)/Acute Exacerbations of Chronic Obstructive Pulmonary Disease (AECOPD)

General Overview of Acute Exacerbations

- An acute sustained worsening of baseline symptoms (cough, sputum, and dyspnea) in those with chronic cough and sputum production (chronic bronchitis) or chronic airflow obstruction (COPD) represents an exacerbation called AECB or AECOPD, respectively.

- Patients with AECOPD can present with purulent or non-purulent exacerbations.

- Since an acute exacerbation may be the first presentation of COPD, spirometry is not useful during exacerbations and should be considered after recovery, to confirm a suspicion of COPD diagnosis.

Treatment of Acute Exacerbations

- Treatment should provide symptomatic relief, prevent loss of lung function that would lead to hospitalization, and lead to re-evaluation of disease to reduce risk of future exacerbations (Balter 2003).

- Remove patients from any sources of irritants (e.g., dust, pollutants, first- and second-hand smoke).

- The goals of pharmacological therapy are to:
  - decrease the work of breathing (bronchodilators)
  - reduce airway inflammation (short-term course of corticosteroids)
  - reduce bacterial burden in the lower airways (antibiotic therapy)
  - treat any accompanying hypoxemia (oxygen therapy)

- For patients with severe exacerbations of COPD and respiratory failure, non-invasive ventilation is an effective therapy that has been shown to reduce mortality.

- Expectorant agents or cough suppressants are of no proven benefit during exacerbations (Balter 2003).

- Provide influenza and pneumococcal vaccinations once recovered.

- For severe exacerbations, oxygen supplementation may be required.

Acute Exacerbations and Role of Antibiotics

- Approximately 50% of AECB/AECOPD are non-infectious (exposure to allergens/irritants e.g., cigarette smoke, dust, cold air, pollution, chemical irritants), while the other 50% are infectious (bacterial, viral).

- Many of the primary viral or non-infectious etiologies cause secondary bacterial infections due to chronic bacterial colonization as a result of airway inflammation.

- A study by Anthonisen et al (1987) categorized acute exacerbations on the existence of specific factors; increased dyspnea, sputum volume and sputum purulence. It was found that exacerbations presenting with at least two of these factors would benefit from treatment with an antibiotic.

- It has also been suggested that antibiotics are warranted in COPD patients presenting with green (purulent) sputum, with an increase from baseline in either dyspnea or cough (Balter 2003; O'Donnell 2003, 2004; Stockley 2000).

Table 12. Pharmacotherapy of COPD: Antibiotic Therapy for AECB / AECOPD[1,2]

Modifying Circumstances	Probabie Organism(s)		Antibiotic Choice(s)	Usual Oral Dosage	Daily Cost
LOW-RISK PATIENTS GROUP 1	H. influenzae S. pneumoniae M. catarrhalis H. species	FIRST LINE	Tetracycline	250-500 mg 4 times daily	$0.08-$0.15
			Doxycycline	100 mg twice daily for first day then 100 mg daily	$0.59
			Amoxicillin	500 mg 3 times daily	$0.60
			TMP/SMX (Cotrimoxazole)	2 tabs or 1 DS tab twice daily	$0.19-$0.24
			Cefuroxime axetil	500 mg twice daily	$4.01
			Cefprozil	500 mg twice daily	$6.00
			Clarithromycin	1000 mg (extended release) daily or 500 mg twice daily	$5.03-$5.92
			Azithromycin	500 mg on first day then 250 mg daily x 4 days	$3.73
		SECOND LINE	Amoxicillin/ Clavulanate	875 mg twice daily or 500 mg 3 times daily	$2.52-$2.80
			Levofloxacin[3,4]	500-750 mg once daily	$3.51-$5.26
			Moxifloxacin[3]	400 mg once daily	$5.01
			Telithromycin[5]	800 mg daily x 5 days	$6.21
HIGH-RISK PATIENTS GROUP 2	H. influenzae S. pneumoniae M. catarrhalis H. species K. pneumoniae	FIRST LINE	Amoxicillin/ Clavulanate	875 mg twice daily or 500 mg 3 times daily	$2.52-$2.80
			Levofloxacin[6]	500-750 mg once daily	$3.51-$5.26
			Moxifloxacin[6]	400 mg once daily	$5.01
PATIENTS AT RISK FOR P. aeruginosa GROUP 3	P. aeruginosa	FIRST LINE	Ciprofloxacin	500-750 mg twice daily	$3.16-$5.95

1) **Risk Stratification (Balter 2003):**

   Low-risk (Group 1) patients have chronic bronchitis defined as having chronic cough and sputum production for at least three months for two consecutive years. They usually have mild to moderate impairment of lung function (FEV_1 > 50% predicted), have fewer than four exacerbations per year and have no significant cardiac disease. Any of the listed antibiotics generally produce good results and the prognosis is excellent.

   High-risk (Group 2) patients may have poor underlying lung function (FEV_1 < 50% predicted) or moderate impairment (FEV_1 between 50% and 60% predicted) but demonstrate significant cardiac disease (ischemic heart disease, congestive heart failure) and/or experience four or more exacerbations a year. They may also have other risk factors including use of supplemental oxygen, chronic use of oral steroids, or antibiotic use in the past 3 months. **High-risk patients who fail to respond to antibiotics usually require admission for intravenous antibiotic combinations.**

   Patients at risk for pseudomonas infection (Group 3) have very poor underlying lung function (FEV_1 < 35% predicted) or multiple risk factors including frequent exacerbations, chronic oral steroid use, and/or FEV_1 < 50% predicted. They produce constant purulent sputum and some may have bronchiectasis.

2) **Patients with a relapse within 3 months of using an antibiotic** (includes macrolides, fluoroquinolones, TMP/SMX, but not penicillins/cephalosporins) should receive an alternative class of antibiotic (McGeer 2004).

3) Due to the importance of the **quinolones** for other indications and concern of developing resistance with overuse, these agents should be held in reserve for severe situations and/or high risk patients (Chen 1999; Balter 2006).

4) **Duration of levofloxacin varies with dose (500 mg daily for 7 days OR 750 mg daily for 5 days).**

5) **Telithromycin is contraindicated in patients who have previous history of hepatitis, jaundice and/or hypersensitivity (especially if associated with the previous use of this drug or macrolides). Telithromycin is also not recommended for patients with myasthenia gravis. Patients should be cautioned about the potential effects of syncope (loss of consciousness) on activities such as driving a vehicle, operating machinery, etc.** Physicians and patients should monitor for signs or symptoms of liver problems (such as fatigue, malaise, anorexia, nausea, jaundice, pruritus, etc). Most post-marketing cases of hepatitis dysfunction were reversible after discontinuation; however, cases of severe hepatotoxicity, including necrosis, hepatitic failure and death have occurred. In some cases liver injury occurred after only a few doses of telithromycin and progressed rapidly **(Clay 2006, Health Canada 2006; Product monograph).**

6) **Fluoroquinolones** may provide better bacterial eradication leading to an accelerated recovery and prolonged disease free intervals (Wilson 2002, 2004; GLOBE and MOSAIC trials).

References: Aaron 2003; Adler 2000; ALF 2003; Anthonisen 1987, 2003; Aubier 2002; Balter 2003, 2006; Bonomo 2002; BTS 2004; Burge 2000; Chen 1999; GOLD 2006; Niewoehner 1999; O'Donnell 2003, 2004; Stockley 2000; Weiss 2002; Wilson 2002, 2004; Zervos 2003; Zhanel 2002.

Adapted from Rosser WW et al. Anti-infective guidelines for community-acquired infections 2005.

Oxygen Therapy in COPD

(ATS/ERS 2005; BTS 2004; GOLD 2006; O'Donnell 2003, 2004; PRODIGY 2006)

Ensuring the patient is receiving optimal medical management is also an important component of evaluation for the need of long-term oxygen therapy.

The risk of progressive hypoxemia is always a concern with COPD patients. Long-term oxygen therapy reduces mortality and increases the life expectancy of COPD patients with chronic hypoxemia.

With longer exposure to supplemental oxygen, there are increased benefits in terms of survival. Long-term continuous oxygen is given for 15 hours/day or more to achieve a saturation of 90% or greater.

The **need** for oxygen therapy should (or can) be assessed in patients with:	• Severe airflow obstruction ($FEV_1 < 30\%$ predicted) • Cyanosis • Polycythemia • Peripheral edema • Raised JVP • Oxygen saturations $\leq 92\%$ on room air
Oxygen therapy is **indicated** in the following situations:	• All patients with stable COPD on optimal doses of medications with $PaO_2 \leq 55$ mmHg or $SaO_2 < 88\%$ • COPD patients with PaO_2 55-59 mmHg or SaO_2 88-90% with concomitant bilateral ankle edema, cor pulmonale, right-sided heart failure, pulmonary hypertension, alterations in mental status or a hematocrit > 56%
Oxygen therapy **may also be considered** in the following situations:	• Desaturation for more than 30% of the time in bed with SaO_2 < 88%, or in the presence of pulmonary hypertension, cor pulmonale or other associated medical conditions that might influence survival • Documented (blinded and repeatable) improvements in dyspnea and exercise performance with oxygen therapy • Short burst therapy to relieve symptoms of severe breathlessness not relieved by other treatments
Oxygen therapy **should not** be used in the following situations:	• Isolated nocturnal desaturations • Patients unwilling to stop smoking

Other Management Issues:
Survival, End Stage COPD & End-of-Life Decision Making in COPD

Survival in COPD

A number of predictive indices exist which estimate the survival of COPD patients based on different variables. Two are noted below as examples, however while applicable to large groups of stable patients, they may not allow for accurate predictions of mortality in individual patients (O'Donnell 2004).

Three Year Survival in COPD (Anthonisen 1986)	
FEV$_1$ % Predicted (post-bronchodilator)	% Surviving at 3 years
> 50%	~ 85%
40-49%	~ 82%
30-39%	~ 73%
< 30%	~ 60%

The BODE index is a multidimensional staging system for COPD that may be better than FEV$_1$ in predicting risk of death. The main variables in this index are BMI (body-mass index), obstruction (FEV$_1$), dyspnea (MMRC = modified MRC scale) and exercise capacity (distance walked over 6 minutes in metres). Refer to Celli (2004) for more details.

Treatment of End-Stage COPD

The treatment of patients with end-stage COPD should follow guidelines based on severity as outlined elsewhere in this document. In addition to optimal pharmacotherapy management of COPD, the following should also be considered:

- Treatment of complications of COPD (e.g., heart failure, pulmonary hypertension)
- Pulmonary rehabilitation and nutritional program to improve overall status
- Long-term oxygen therapy if patient meets criteria
- Potential surgical intervention

End-of-Life Decision Making (O'Donnell 2004)

COPD is a progressive, disabling disease that eventually leads to premature death for many patients. It is important, therefore, to anticipate the eventual need for end-of-life decision making for these patients. Unfortunately, discussions about end-of-life issues often do not meet patient expectations, occur very late and in unsuitable settings (e.g., ICU). The important skills that patients think physicians need in order to provide end-of-life care include: the ability to provide emotional support, to communicate, to be accessible and to provide continuity of care. It is important for physicians to provide information in five areas; diagnosis and disease process, treatment, prognosis, what dying might be like, and advance care planning.

APPENDICES

Appendix A

Measurement of Lung Function
(Lowry 1998; BTS 2004)

Definitions

Term	Definition	Comments	Normal Range
FVC Forced Vital Capacity [Litres]	• Maximum volume of air exhaled using maximal effort following maximal inspiration	• Most useful measurement for diagnosing and following restrictive pulmonary diseases	• 80-120% of the predicted value
FEV$_1$ Forced expiratory volume in one second [Litres]	• Maximum volume of air exhaled during the first second of a forced expiratory manoeuvre	• Most important measurement for following obstructive pulmonary disease • Determines the severity of airways obstruction	• 80-120% of the predicted value • Normal rate of decline due to aging ≈ 30 mL per year
FEV$_1$ / FVC ratio		• Used to assess airflow limitation	• Normally greater than 0.75 to 0.80 and possibly greater than 0.90 in children. Ratio < 0.7 indicates an obstructive disorder in middle-aged adults
PEF Peak expiratory flow [L/sec or L/min]	• The highest rate of expiratory flow achieved using maximal forced effort, following maximal inspiration	• Peak flow meters are useful for home monitoring of patients with asthma • May be misleading in COPD	• < 80% of patient's personal best suggests obstruction • < 50% of an asthma patient's personal best indicates an acute asthma attack

Differentiating Available Tests

Differentiating	Measuring	Comments
Spirometry	• Gives a measure of airflow limitation and reversibility • Typical measurements include FVC, FEV$_1$, and FEV$_1$/FVC	• Often done as an outpatient, in the Emergency Department, at hospital pulmonary function laboratory, or at the bedside
Flow Volume Loop	• Often included in the Spirometry report • Can be very helpful when differentiating atypical patterns of obstruction or restriction	• Can suggest rare cases of fixed upper or lower airway obstruction
Pulmonary Function Tests (PFTs)	• Combination of Spirometry (pre- and post-β$_2$-agonist) **and Carbon Monoxide Diffusion capacity and lung volumes**	• Performed in a Pulmonary Functionary laboratory, which is often hospital-based • **Not necessary for the routine diagnosis and management of Asthma and COPD**

Appendix A *(continued)*

Factors that Influence Normal Values of Pulmonary Function

- Most spirometers factor in gender, height, age, and race when calculating the predicted FEV_1 and FVC.

- However, when faced with abnormal FEV_1 values, physicians should consider the following factors in their treatment management plans:

Factor	Influence	Comment
Gender	Lung volumes in males are generally larger than in females	
Race	Non-Caucasians may have smaller lung volumes and possibly lower predicted values	Appropriate predictive equations for FEV_1 and FVC should be established for each patient
Age	Lung volumes decrease with age	Be careful interpreting data from very young (< 20 years) or very old (> 70 years) patients when using prediction equations
Height	Based on prediction equations, patients with "extremes of height" may be misinterpreted as having abnormal pulmonary functions	Use measured, rather than stated patient height
Posture	Volume measurements may be decreased with supine position	Ensure upright posture during spirometry testing

Appendix B

Tests for Diagnosing and Monitoring Asthma
(Boulet 1999; GINA 2006)

In children (over 5 years of age) and adults, objective measures are used in confirming the diagnosis of asthma, assessing the severity and monitoring the course of the illness. The availability and utility of these tests vary in the family practice setting but are included for reference purposes:

Spirometry	**Recommended method of measuring airflow limitation and reversibility to establish a diagnosis of asthma. The degree of reversibility in FEV_1 that supports a diagnosis of asthma is generally:** • **$\geq$ 12% (preferably 15%) (and $\geq$ 200 mL) improvement in FEV_1 from the baseline 15 minutes after using a short-acting inhaled β_2-agonist.** However, most asthma patients will not exhibit reversibility at each assessment, particularly those on treatment, and the test therefore lacks sensitivity. Repeated testing at different visits is advised.
Peak Expiratory Flow (PEF)	**Not preferred method** for establishing diagnosis of asthma. PEF measurements are not interchangeable with the more sensitive and reliable FEV_1 measurements. PEF may underestimate the degree of airflow limitation, especially when airflow limitation and gas trapping are worsening. When spirometry is not available a diagnosis of asthma is suggested **when:** • **A 60L/min (or 20% or more of pre-bronchodilator PEF) improvement after inhalation of a bronchodilator, or diurnal PEF variability $\geq$ 20% (with twice daily readings, more than 10%).** • **For monitoring/improving asthma control:** Usually measurements are taken first thing in the morning (before any treatment and values are near their lowest) and last thing at night. Compare PEF measurements (using patients own meter) to patient's own previous best measurements.
Airway Hyper-responsiveness Methacholine Challenge Test	**A methacholine challenge test** is useful to measure airway hyperresponsiveness when the diagnosis of asthma is in doubt (e.g., suggestive history, but normal spirometry at rest). This is performed in specialized pulmonary function laboratories.
Measurement of Allergic Status	**Measurement of allergic status** is an important consideration because of the strong association between asthma and allergies. Consider an eosinophilic count, serum IgE, and/or allergen skin testing in patients not responding to standard asthma therapy.

Appendix C

Occupational Asthma
(Newman 2004; www.bohrf.org.uk)

- Occupational asthma is estimated to account for 9-15% of all adult-onset asthma.

- Occupational asthma tends to have a poor prognosis unless identified and managed early.

- Approximately one third of workers with occupational asthma are unemployed up to 6 years after diagnosis and suffer financially.

- The most frequently reported agents include isocyanates, flour and grain dust, colophony and fluxes, latex, animals, aldehydes and wood dust.

- In all new cases of adult asthma consider the possibility of occupational asthma especially in individuals with high risk occupations (e.g., animal handlers, bakers and pastry makers, chemical workers, food processing workers, nurses, paint sprayers, timber workers, and welders).

- Individuals presenting with asthma symptoms or rhinitis should be asked about their job and the substances with which they work. Rhinitis occurring in patients in high risk occupations might signal an increased risk of developing occupational asthma within 12 months of the onset of rhinitis.

- Improvement in symptoms (wheeze and/or shortness of breath) when away from work has been shown to be a good indicator that occupational asthma may exist. Some helpful questions to ask the patient include: When did the symptoms start? Do their symptoms vary when not a work? Do their symptoms improve when away from work, especially during long holidays?

- Objective investigations help confirm the diagnosis of occupational asthma (e.g., serial PEF, challenge testing) and referral to a specialist is useful, especially if they fall into one of the high risk occupations.

- The primary care physician may be able to initiate some of these objective investigations, such as serial monitoring of peak expiratory flow.

It is recommended that the patient be referred early to a respirologist for formal evaluation and documentation while still employed.

Classification and Management of Work-Related Asthma
(Boulet 1999; Newman 2004; Nicholson 2005; Tarlo 1998, 2003, 2006)

Work-related Asthma	Notes	Management
Occupational Asthma **Sensitizer-induced** **(Immunological)**	• More common type of occupational asthma (90% of cases) • Caused by an IgE-mediated or other immune response to specific workplace agents • Once a person has been sensitized, even exposure to extremely low quantities will exacerbate the asthma	• Treatment of asthma • Referral to a specialist • Complete removal of patient from future exposure to workplace sensitizer
Occupational Asthma **Irritant-induced** **(non-immunological)**	• Less common form of occupational asthma (about 7% of cases) • Occurs after accidental exposure to very high inhaled concentrations of workplace irritant	• Treatment of asthma • Modification of work environment to reduce exposure to aggravating irritants • Reduce risk of future accidental exposures affecting same worker or others
Aggravation of Pre-existing or Coincidental Asthma	• Aggravation of pre-existing asthma due to workplace exposures to potential irritants • More likely to occur in patients with moderate or severe forms of asthma and in those not receiving optimal treatment	• Optimization of asthma management • If needed, reduction of workplace exposures to respiratory irritants • Patient may be able to stay in same job, but requires reduction in exposure to triggers

Appendix C *(continued)*

Occupational Asthma: Workplace Sensitizers

Examples of workplace sensitizers to which workers in various professions may be exposed* (Tarlo 2003; GINA 2006)	
Occupation	**Potential sensitizers**
Automotive Workers	• Diisocyanates or epoxy compounds in spray paints • Diisocyanates in manufacture of rigid or flexible polyurethane foam and glues
Bakers and Pastry Makers	• Flour, amylase
Cleaners and Laboratory Workers	• Enzymes or cleaning agents • Latex in gloves
Electronic Workers	• Colophony (pine resin) or amines in soldering flux • Acrylic glues
Farmers, Gardeners	• Soybean dust; animal, plant, insect and fungal allergens; dairy farmers (storage mites); Poultry farmers exposed to mites, droppings, feathers
Food Processors and Animal Workers	• Egg processors exposed to egg proteins; fish food processors exposed to midges, parasites, shellfish amylase; veterinarians exposed to dander, urine proteins; Others substances include coffee bean dust, tea, meat tenderizer, psyllium, pancreatic enzymes, papain
Hairdressers, Beauticians	• Persulphate in hair bleaches, *Para*-phenylenediamine in hair dyes
Health Care Workers	• Natural rubber latex in gloves • Glutaraldehyde used in sterilization of endoscopy equipment and development of x-ray film • Penicillin and other aerosolized or powdered medications (e.g., psyllium)
Plastics and Rubber Industry	• Diisocyanates, acrylates, anhydrides, tetramines, formaldehyde, diamines
Welders and Other Metal Workers	• Metal dusts or fumes (e.g., nickel, cobalt, chromium, platinum, vanadium) • Coolants containing pine products or other sensitizers
Woodworkers	• Dusts from red cedar and other woods • Phenol formaldehyde resins in particle board • Diisocyanates in glues

* More than 300 substances have been associated with occupational asthma (See http://www.remcomp.com/asmanet/asmapro/agents.htm for a comprehensive list)

Appendix D

Pharmacotherapy - Other Options*

Class	Medication	Common Dosage Forms and Usual Daily Dosage
Short-acting β₂-agonists (SABA) (in alphabetical order)	**Fenoterol hydrobromide** (Berotec®)	**Inhalation solution via nebulizer: 1 mg/mL** Adults: 0.5-1 mg/dose up to 2.5 mg/dose as needed; May be repeated every 6 hours if needed Children ≥ 12 years: 0.1-1 mg/dose; May be repeated every 6 hours if needed
	Salbutamol sulfate (Ventolin®, Airomir®, generics)	**Diskus®: 200 µg/blister for oral inhalation** Adults and children > 4 years: 200 µg 3-4 times daily as needed; May be repeated if needed; Maximum of 800 µg/day **Respirator solution via nebulizer: 0.5, 1, or 2 mg/mL nebules; 5 mg/mL inhalation solution** Adults: 2.5-5 mg as needed; May be repeated 4 times/day if needed Children: 0.05-0.15 mL/kg/dose as needed. May be repeated 4 times daily if needed **For severe refractory cases, a single dose of salbutamol inhalation solution may be increased to 5 mg** **Oral liquid: 0.4 mg/mL** Adults and children > 12 years: 2-4 mg 3-4 times/day Children 6-12 years: 2 mg 3-4 times/day Children 2-6 years: 0.1 mg/kg 3-4 times/day **Oral tablets: 2 mg, 4 mg** Adults: 2-4 mg 3-4 times/day; May increase to 8 mg 4 times/day Children > 12 years: 2-4 mg 3-4 times/day Children 6-12 years: 2 mg 3-4 times/day
Short-acting Inhaled Anticholinergic	**Ipratropium bromide** (Atrovent®)	**Inhalation solution via nebulizer: 125 or 250 µg/mL** Adults: 250-500 µg, then every 4-6 hours as needed Children 5-12 years: 125-250 µg, then every 4-6 hours as needed Daily doses exceeding 2 mg in adults should be given under medical supervision.

* Consult latest product monographs for current availability and dosing.

Appendix D *(continued)*

Pharmacotherapy - Other Options*

Class	Medication	Common Dosage Forms and Usual Daily Dosage	
Combination Therapy Short-acting β_2-agonist + Short-acting Inhaled Anticholinergic	**Ipratropium bromide** + **Fenoterol hydrobromide** (Duovent® UDV)	**Inhalation solution via nebulizer: 0.5 mg ipratropium and 1.25 mg fenoterol per 4 mL in isotonic saline (plastic unit-dose vials)** Adults and children ≥ 12 years: 4 mL via nebulizer. May be repeated after 6 hours if necessary	
	Ipratropium bromide + **Salbutamol sulfate** (Combivent®)	**Inhalation solution via nebulizer: 0.5 mg ipratropium and 2.5 mg salbutamol per 2.5 mL unit-dose vial** 2.5 mL/dose; May be repeated every 6 hours if needed	
Inhaled Cortico-steriods (ICS)	**Budesonide** (Pulmicort®)	**Nebuamp via nebulizer: 0.125, 0.25, or 0.5 mg/mL**	
		Adults:	0.5 mg-1 mg twice daily. Maximum of 4 mg/day
		Children > 12 years:	0.5-1 mg twice daily
		Children 3 months - 12 years:	0.25-0.5 mg twice daily. Maximum of 1 mg twice daily

* Consult latest product monographs for current availability and dosing.

Appendix D *(continued)*

Available Drugs, Dosage Form and Strengths
(Consult latest product monographs for current availability)

Inhaled Bronchodilators

Class	Generic Name	Common Brand Name	Devices and Strengths Available	
ANTI-CHOLINERGICS	Ipratropium bromide	Atrovent®	Atrovent® HFA pMDI (200 doses)	20 µg / inhalation
			Inhalation solution	125 µg/mL; 2 mL plastic single-use vials
				250 µg/mL; 1 and 2 mL plastic single-use vials, 20 mL amber glass bottles
	Tiotropium bromide monohydrate	Spiriva®	HandiHaler® inhalation device (cartons of 10 or 30 capsules)	18 µg capsule for inhalation
SHORT-ACTING INHALED β₂-AGONISTS	Fenoterol hydrobromide	Berotec®	pMDI (200 doses)	100 µg / inhalation
			Inhalation solution (via nebulizer)	1 mg/mL; 20 mL amber glass bottles
	Salbutamol sulfate	Ventolin®	Ventolin® HFA (200 doses)	100 µg / inhalation
			Respirator solution (via nebulizer)	0.5, 1, or 2 mg/mL; 2.5 mL nebules
				5 mg/mL; 10 mL stock bottles
			Diskus® (60 doses)	200 µg blister for inhalation
		Airomir®	pMDI (100 or 200 doses)	100 µg / inhalation
	Terbutaline sulfate	Bricanyl®	Turbuhaler® DPI (50 or 200 doses)	0.5 mg / inhalation
LONG-ACTING INHALED β₂-AGONISTS	Formoterol fumarate dihydrate	Oxeze®	Turbuhaler® DPI (60 doses)	6 or 12 µg / inhalation
	Formoterol fumarate	Foradil®	Aerolizer™ inhalation device (cartons of 60 capsules)	12 µg capsule for inhalation using Aerolizer™ inhaler
	Salmeterol xinafoate	Serevent®	Diskus® (60 doses)	50 µg / inhalation
			Diskhaler® (cartons of 15 disks; 4 blisters/disk)	50 µg blister for inhalation
			pMDI (60 or 120 doses)	25 µg / inhalation

Inhaled Sodium Cromoglycate

Class	Generic Name	Common Brand Name	Devices and Strengths Available	
Inhaled Sodium Cromoglycate	Sodium cromoglycate	generics	Inhalation solution (via nebulizer)	10 mg/mL; 2 mL ampules

Appendix D *(continued)*

Inhaled Corticosteroids

Class	Generic Name	Common Brand Name	Devices and Strengths Available	
INHALED CORTICOSTEROIDS	Beclomethasone dipropionate	Qvar®	pMDI (100 or 200 doses)	50 or 100 µg / inhalation
	Budesonide	Pulmicort®	Turbuhaler® DPI (200 doses)	100, 200, or 400 µg / inhalation
			Nebuamp® (via nebulizer)	0.125, 0.25, or 0.5 mg/mL; 2 mL ampuls
	Ciclesonide	Alvesco®	pMDI (120 doses)	100 or 200 µg / inhalation
	Fluticasone propionate	Flovent®	pMDI (60 or 100 doses)	50 µg / inhalation (120 doses) 50, 125, or 250 µg / inhalation
			Diskus® (60 blisters)	50, 100, 250, or 500 µg / inhalation

Inhaled Combination Preparations

Class	Generic Name	Common Brand Name	Devices and Strengths Available	
Combination Anticholinergic and Short-Acting β₂-Agonist	Ipratropium bromide + salbutamol sulfate	Combivent®	Inhalation solution (via nebulizer)	0.5 mg ipratropium and 2.5 mg salbutamol per 2.5 mL unit-dose vial
	Ipratropium bromide + Fenoterol hydrobromide	Duovent® UDV	Inhalation solution (via nebulizer)	0.5 mg ipratropium and 1.25 mg fenoterol per 4 mL plastic single-use vials
Combination Long-Acting β₂-Agonist and Inhaled Corticosteroid	Salmeterol xinafoate + Fluticasone propionate	Advair®	pMDI (120 doses)	25 µg salmeterol per inhalation and 125 or 250 µg fluticasone per inhalation
			Diskus® (60 doses)	50 µg salmeterol and 100, 250, or 500 µg fluticasone per blister
	Formoterol fumarate dihydrate + Budesonide	Symbicort®	Turbuhaler® DPI (60 or 120 doses)	6 µg formoterol and 100 or 200 µg budesonide per inhalation (breath activated dry powder inhaler for oral inhalation)

For further information about inhalation devices, please refer to the
RxFiles (http://www.rxfiles.ca)

II) Oral Bronchodilators

Formulation	Generic Name	Common Brand Name	Devices and Strengths Available
Oral Tablets	Salbutamol	generics	2 mg tablet 4 mg tablet
Oral Liquids	Salbutamol	Ventolin® Oral Liquid and generics	0.4 mg/mL; 250 mL bottles

Appendix D *(continued)*

III) Leukotriene Receptor Antagonists

Formulation	Generic Name	Common Brand Name	Devices and Strengths Available
Oral Tablets	Montelukast	Singulair®	4 mg and 5 mg chewable tablet 10 mg tablet, and 4 mg oral granules
	Zafirlukast	Accolate®	20 mg tablet

IV) IgE Monoclonal Antibodies

Formulation	Generic Name	Common Brand Name	Devices and Strengths Available
Sterile Powder for Reconstitution Subcutaneous Injection	Omalizumab	Xolair®	150 mg vial

V) Xanthine Preparations

Theophylline

Formulation	Generic Name	Common Brand Name	Strengths Available	Unit Cost
Oral Extended Release	Theophylline	Somophyllin-12®	50 mg LA capsule	$0.17
		Uniphyl®	400 mg SR tablet	$0.46
			600 mg SR tablet	$0.55
		Novo®-Theophyl SR	100 mg SR tablet	$0.13
			200 mg SR tablet	$0.14
			300 mg SR tablet	$0.14
		Apo®-Theo LA	100 mg SR tablet	$0.13
			200 mg SR tablet	$0.14
			300 mg SR tablet	$0.14
Elixir	Theophylline	PMS-Theophylline oral liquid	80 mg/15 mL	$0.07 per 15 mL
		Theolair™ oral liquid (alcohol-free)	80 mg/15 mL	$0.07 per 15 mL

Oxtriphylline

Formulation	Generic Name	Common Brand Name	Strengths Available	Unit Cost
Oral Tablets	Oxtriphylline	Apo®-Oxtriphylline	100 mg tablet (= 64 mg anhydrous theophylline)	$0.02
			200 mg tablet (= 128 mg anhydrous theophylline)	$0.02
			300 mg tablet (= 192 mg anhydrous theophylline)	$0.03
Elixir	Oxtriphylline	Choledyl™ PMS-Oxtriphylline	100 mg/5 mL (= 64 mg theophylline)	$0.11 per 5 mL

Aminophylline

Formulation	Generic Name	Common Brand Name	Strengths Available	Unit Cost
Oral Tablets	Aminophylline	generics	100 mg tablet	
Oral Extended Release	Aminophylline	Phyllocontin®	225 mg SR tablet (= 182.25 mg anhydrous theophylline)	$0.20
			350 mg SR tablet (= 283.5 mg anhydrous theophylline)	$025

...dix E

Proposed Dose Equivalencies for Inhaled Corticosteroids in Asthma
(Becker 2005; Boulet 1999; Lemière 2004)

Inhaled corticosteroids are used for the long-term management of asthma; they are recommended as *first-line agents* in asthma control (Becker 2005).

Generic Name	Common Brand Name	Dose µg/day		
		Low	Medium	High
Beclomethasone dipropionate	Qvar® pMDI	≤ 250	251 - 500	> 500
Beclomethasone dipropionate + spacer	Qvar® pMDI	≤ 500	501 - 1000	> 1000
Budesonide	Pulmicort® Turbuhaler®	≤ 400	401 - 800	> 800
Budesonide solution or wet nebulisation	Pulmicort® Nebuamp®	≤ 1000	1001 - 2000	> 2000
Ciclesonide	Alvesco® pMDI	≤ 200	201 - 400	> 400
Fluticasone propionate + spacer	Flovent® pMDI	≤ 250	251 - 500	> 500
Fluticasone propionate	Flovent® Diskus®	≤ 250	251 - 500	> 500

Appendix F

Pharmacotherapy: Theophylline in Asthma and COPD

- Oral theophylline offers the patient advantages in terms of ease of administration and better patient compliance with a once or twice daily sustained-release product

- Long-acting products have also been shown to reduce overnight declines in FEV_1 and morning respiratory symptoms, but this benefit may be more safely achieved by LABAs

---

Role of theophylline in Asthma

Theophylline is generally considered a 3rd line agent in asthma, after inhaled corticosteroids, LABAs, and LTRAs. It may be beneficial to add theophylline therapy to improve control in patients who are prescribed high doses of ICS or who experience nocturnal symptoms.

Role of theophylline in COPD

Theophylline may be considered as adjunctive therapy for those COPD patients whose conditions are difficult to treat with inhaled bronchodilators alone. Although theophylline is a weaker bronchodilator than the inhaled anticholinergic or β_2-agonist medications, it may provide additional benefits in improving dyspnea, exertional endurance, nocturnal symptoms and quality of life for some patients with COPD. These beneficial effects on symptoms are thought to be due to non-bronchodilating properties of theophylline.

- The **therapeutic range** of theophylline has conventionally been regarded as 55-110 µmol/L, but recent data indicates beneficial effects at concentrations below the upper limit of this range

- Hence, current strategies aim to achieve lower serum theophylline levels (55-85 µmol/L and 28-55 µmol/L, in COPD and asthma, respectively), which are associated with fewer side effects

- The **maximum safe dose** is reflected by a steady-state peak serum concentration obtained 8-12 hours after a once-a-day preparation or 4-6 hours after a twice-a-day preparation (time to steady state may vary with different formulations)

- A trough serum concentration obtained prior to the next dose may be helpful in assuring therapeutic theophylline concentrations are being maintained

Theophylline serum levels are affected by many medications:

- Cimetidine, erythromycin, ciprofloxacin, verapamil, fluvoxamine, and pharmacologically similar agents will increase serum levels

- Smoking, phenytoin, carbamazepine, and rifampin will decrease levels

Dose equivalencies for xanthine derivatives

Theophylline anhydrous	Aminophylline anhydrous	Oxtriphylline	Theophylline sodium glycinate
100 mg	118 mg	156 mg	200 mg

Please refer to Appendix D for available strengths of xanthine preparations

Appendix G

Adverse Drug Effects of Asthma/COPD Medications

Drug	Common Side Effects/Drug Interactions
Inhaled β_2-agonists	<ul><li>Tachycardia, palpitations, tremor and prolongation of QT interval.</li><li>Repeated high doses can cause hypokalemia, increase myocardial oxygen demands.</li><li>Oral or topical nonselective beta blockers can precipitate bronchospasm in asthmatic patients and decrease the bronchodilating effect of β_2-agonists; they are relatively contraindicated in patients with asthma (but not for COPD).</li><li>Long-acting inhaled β_2-agonists should not be used alone.</li></ul>
Inhaled Corticosteroids	<ul><li>Oral candidiasis and dysphonia. Other risk factors for developing candidiasis include concomitant use of antibiotics/systemic steroids (common during exacerbations) and presence of xerostomia (often induced by systemic anticholinergic agents/antidepressants). Reduce occurrence of candidiasis by reducing total daily dose, dose frequency and oropharyngeal deposition by using a spacer and rinsing mouth after each dose.</li><li>Higher doses of ICS associated with suppression of hypothalamic-pituitary-adrenal (HPA) axis. No significant difference was reported between inhaled ciclesonide and placebo on HPA function and serum cortisol levels (Derom 2005).</li><li>In children, a reduction in growth velocity may occur in the first year of treatment with inhaled corticosteroids. Prospective studies show that children treated with moderate doses of ICS for long periods of time attain their predicted adult height (Becker 2005).</li><li>Ocular issues. Avoid contact of pressurized inhaler contents with eyes. Measure intraocular pressures within a few days of initiating therapy in patients with a personal or family history of glaucoma and monitor at appropriate intervals. This is particularly important in patients on high dose inhaled corticosteroids. Routine ophthalmologic surveillance for posterior subcapsular cataract is not required for patients on inhaled corticosteroid.</li><li>Osteoporosis. Elderly patients and postmenopausal women maintained on oral corticosteroids for prolonged periods should be assessed for osteoporosis. (Naganathan et al, 2000). High doses of inhaled beclomethasone do not usually result in significant osteoporotic effects unless other risk factors are present. Bone Mineral Density should be obtained in patients maintained on high ICS doses or those with $\geq$ 1 risk factor for osteoporosis.</li><li>Skin bruising and thinning have been reported.</li><li>Use with itraconazole or ritonavir may increase risk of developing Cushing's syndrome.</li><li>Myopathy has been reported in children receiving high doses of fluticasone.</li></ul>
Oral Corticosteroids	<ul><li>With short-term use: mood changes, glucose intolerance.</li><li>With long-term use: weight gain, hypertension, bone demineralization leading to osteoporosis, cataracts, immunosuppression, thin skin, avascular necrosis of the hip, and decreased linear growth in children.</li></ul>
Leukotriene Receptor Antagonists	<ul><li>Churg-Strauss vasculitis has been associated with LTRA use, but may not be directly related.</li><li>Rare reports of hepatotoxicity.</li><li>Zafirlukast absorption is decreased by food (take 1 hr before or 2 hrs after meals); it may decrease metabolism of drugs such as warfarin, phenytoin, carbamazepine, and cyclosporine; monitor if corticosteroids are being withdrawn.</li></ul>

Appendix G *(continued)*

Adverse Drug Effects of Asthma/COPD Medications

Drug	Common Side Effects/Drug Interactions
Sodium Cromoglycate	• Dryness, throat irritation.
Theophylline	• At serum concentrations higher than 110 µmol/L, higher frequency of: nausea, nervousness, headache, and insomnia. • At higher serum concentrations: vomiting, hypokalemia, hyperglycemia, tachycardia, cardiac arrhythmias, tremor, neuromuscular irritability, and seizures. • Many potential drug interactions.
Ipratropium Bromide or Tiotropium	• Dry mouth, pharyngeal irritation, urinary retention, and increases in intraocular pressure. • Should be used with caution in patients with glaucoma and in those with prostatic hypertrophy or bladder neck obstruction. • Ipratropium pMDI (not HFA) should be avoided in those with allergy to peanuts.
Omalizumab	• Anaphylaxis or anaphylactoid reaction have been reported. • Long-term adverse consequences presently unknown. • Association with tumours has been reported.

Appendix H

Safety of Medications during Pregnancy[1,2]
(ACOG & ACCA 2000; BTS 2005; NAEPP 2004)

Benefits of continuing these agents in patients with moderate-to-severe asthma who are well controlled may outweigh the risks of stopping therapy

Drug Class	Pregnancy Risk Classification		Notes
Inhaled corticosteroids (ICS)	beclomethasone	C	• Use of ICS is normal during pregnancy (BTS 2005). Data from pregnant patients suggest these agents do not increase the risk of adverse outcomes
	budesonide	B	
	ciclesonide	C	• Drugs of choice in pregnant patients with at least mild symptoms of asthma
	fluticasone	C	• Budesonide has been shown to be safe when used during pregnancy, and should be considered if treatment is to be initiated during pregnancy
			• Patients with controlled asthma using another ICS need not to switch to budesonide
Short-acting β₂-agonists	fenoterol	B	• 2 recently published studies have reported that salbutamol is safe
	terbutaline	B	
	salbutamol	C	• SABAs preferred over long-acting agents
Long-acting β₂-agonists	formoterol	C	• No human data published
	salmeterol	C	• Short-acting agents are preferred when initiating therapy
			• Long-acting agents should not be used as monotherapy
Short-acting Anticholinergics	ipratropium	B	• No published data in pregnant patients
			• Animal studies suggest they are safe agents
Long-acting Anticholinergics	tiotropium	X	
Leukotriene receptor antagonists	montelukast	B	• No human studies available. Animal studies did not find any birth defects
	zafirlukast	B	• Initiating treatment with these agents during pregnancy is not recommended
			• May be considered in patients with refractory symptoms who preferentially responded to these agents prior to becoming pregnant
Theophylline-containing products	aminophylline	C	• There are no controlled data in human pregnancy
	oxtriphylline	C	• It has been recommended that theophylline containing preparations should only be used during pregnancy when there are no alternatives and benefit outweighs risk
	theophylline	C	
Oral corticosteroids	prednisone	C	• Prednisone has not been formally assigned to a pregnancy category by the FDA. However prednisolone (its active metabolite), has been assigned to pregnancy category C
			• Benefits outweigh risks in the treatment of severe asthma exacerbations
			• It is recommended that pregnant women taking oral/systemic corticosteroids have a level 2 (very detailed) ultrasound done at 16-18 weeks to detect structural abnormalities, assess severity of abnormalities, and determine if/when surgery will be needed
			• Use of oral/systemic corticosteroids in the first 12 weeks of pregnancy is associated with a small increase in the risk of cleft palate (risk is 2 in 1000 compared to normal incidence of 1 in 1000)
			• Conflicting data; causality not established

Appendix H *(Continued)*

Safety of Medications during Pregnancy
(ACOG & ACCA 2000; NAEPP 2004; BTS 2005)

Antibiotics	Pregnancy Risk Classifications
Amoxicillin	B
Amoxicillin / Clavulanate	B
Azithromycin	B
Cefuroxime	B
Cefprozil	B
Ciprofloxacin	C
Clarithromycin	C
Cotrimoxazole	C
Doxycycline	D
Gatifloxacin	C
Levofloxacin	C
Moxifloxacin	C
Telithromycin	C
Tetracycline	D

1) Labeling of some prescription drugs includes information about the level of risk for the fetus and the extent of caution necessary in their use. The FDA has established five categories (A, B, C, D, and X) to indicate a drug's potential for causing teratogenicity. This format was first announced in the September 1979 FDA Drug Bulletin. Because of labeling revisions, many products now use this format.

2) Use of asthma medications while breastfeeding can be continued as normal, following manufacturers' recommendations (BTS 2005).

US FDA Pregnancy Category Definitions	
A	Controlled studies in women fail to demonstrate a risk to the fetus in the first trimester (and there is no evidence of a risk in later trimesters), and the possibility of fetal harm appears remote.
B	Either animal-reproduction studies have not demonstrated a fetal risk but there are no controlled studies in pregnant women or animal-reproduction studies have shown adverse effect (other than a decrease in fertility) that was not confirmed in controlled studies in women in the first trimester (and there is no evidence of a risk in later trimesters).
C	Either studies in animals have revealed adverse effects on the fetus (teratogenic or embryocidal or other) and there are no controlled studies in women or studies in women and animals are not available. Drugs should be given only if the potential benefit justifies the potential risk to the fetus.
D	There is positive evidence of human fetal risk, but the benefits from use in pregnant women may be acceptable despite the risk (e.g., if the drug is needed in a life-threatening situation or for a serious disease for which safer drugs cannot be used or are ineffective).
X	Studies in animals or human beings have demonstrated fetal abnormalities or there is evidence of fetal risk based on human experience or both, and the risk of the use of the drug in pregnant women clearly outweighs any possible benefit. The drug is contraindicated in women who are or may become pregnant.

Bibliography

1) AAAAI (The American Academy of Allergy, Asthma & Immunology, Inc). Attaining optimal asthma control: A practice parameter. J Allergy Clin Immunol 2005;116:S3-11.

2) AAAAI (The American Academy of Allergy, Asthma & Immunology, Inc). Pediatric asthma: Promoting best practice. Guide for managing asthma in children. Milwaukee. 2004. Available at: http://www.aaaai.org/members/resources/initiatives/pediatricasthma.stm.

3) Aaron SD, Vandemheen KL, Hebert P et al. Outpatient oral prednisone after emergency department treatment of chronic obstructive pulmonary disease. N Engl J Med 2003;348:2618-25.

4) ACOG & ACAAI (American College of Obstetricians and Gynecologists (ACOG) and the American College of Allergy, Asthma and Immunology). The use of newer asthma and allergy medications during pregnancy. Ann Allergy Asthma Immunol 2000;84:475-80.

5) Adler JL, Jannetti W, Schneider D et al. Phase III, randomized, double blind study of clarithromycin extended release and immediate release formulation in the treatment of patients with acute exacerbation of chronic bronchitis. Clinical Therapeutics 2000;22:1410-20.

6) Agertoft L, Pedersen S. Effect of long-term treatment with inhaled budesonide on height in children with asthma. N Engl J Med 2000;343:1064-9.

7) Albert RK, Martin TR, Lewis SW. Controlled clinical trial of methylprednisolone in patients with chronic bronchitis and acute respiratory insufficiency. Ann Intern Med 1980;92:753-8.

8) (ALF, 2006) Australian Lung Foundation and the Thoracic Society of Australia and New Zealand. The COPDX Plan: Australian and New Zealand guidelines for the management of chronic obstructive pulmonary disease. Australian Lung Foundation; 2006.

9) Alfageme I, Vazquez R, Reyes N et al. Clinical efficacy of anti-pneumococcal vaccination in patients with COPD. Thorax 2006;61:189-95.

10) Almqvist C, Egmar AC, van Hage-Hamsten M et al. Heredity, pet ownership, and confounding control in a population-based birth cohort. J Allergy Clin Immunol 2003;111:800-6.

11) Anthonisen NR, Connett JE, Kiley JP et al. Effects of smoking intervention and the use of anticholinergic bronchodilator on the rate of decline of FEV1. The lung health study. JAMA 1994;272:1497-505.

12) Anthonisen NR, Connett JE, Murrary RP, for the Lung Health Study research group. Smoking and lung function of lung health study participants after 11 years. Am J Respir Crit Care Med 2002;166:675-9.

13) Anthonisen NR, Manfred J, Warren CPW et al. Antibiotic therapy in exacerbations of chronic obstructive pulmonary disease. Ann Intern Med 1987;106:196-204.

14) Anthonisen NR, Wright EC, and the IPPB Trial Group. Bronchodilator response in chronic obstructive pulmonary disease. Am Rev Respir Dis 1986;133:814-19.

15) Anthonisen NR, Wright EC, Hodgkin JE et al. Prognosis in chronic obstructive pulmonary disease. Am Rev Respir Dis 1986;133:14-20.

16) Anthonisen NR, Connett JE, Murray RP, for the Lung Health Study Research Group. Smoking and lung function of lung health study participants after 11 years. Am J Respir Crit Care Med 2002;166:675-9.

17) (ATS) American Thoracic Society/ European Respiratory Society. Standards for the diagnosis and management of patients with COPD. New York: American Thoracic Society;2005.

18) (ATS) American Thoracic Society/ European Respiratory Society. Statement on pulmonary rehabilitation. Am J Resp Crit Care 2006;173:1390-1413.

19) Aubier M, Aldons PM, Leak A et al. Telithromycin is as effective as amoxicillin/clavulanate in acute exacerbations of chronic bronchitis. Respir Med 2002;96:862-71.

20) Balter MS, Hyland RH, Low DE et al. Recommendations on the management of chronic bronchitis: a practical guide for Canadian physicians. Can Med Assoc J 1994;151:5-23.

21) Balter MS, La Forge J, Low DE et al. Canadian guidelines for the management of acute exacerbations of chronic bronchitis. Can Resp J 2003;10(suppl B):3B-32.

22) Balter MS. Personal Communication. Mount Sinai Hospital: Toronto. 2006.

23) Balter MS, Weiss K. Treating acute exacerbations of chronic bronchitis and community-acquired pneumonia. Can Fam Physician 2006;52:1236-42.

24) Beach J, Rowe BH, Blitz S et al. Diagnosis and management of work-related asthma. Publication NO. 06-E003-1. Rockville, MD: Agency for Healthcare Research and Quality. October 2005.

25) Becker A, Watson W, Ferguson A et al. The Canadian asthma primary prevention study: outcomes at 2 years of age. J Allergy Clin Immunol 2004;113:650-6.

26) Becker A, Lemière C, Bérubé D et al. Summary of recommendations from the Canadian Asthma Consensus Guidelines, 2003. CMAJ 2005;173:S3-11.

27) Becker A, Bérubé D, Chad Z et al. Canadian pediatric asthma consensus guidelines, 2003 (updated to December 2004). CMAJ 2005;173:S12-55.

28) Bergeron C, Boulet L-P, and Hamid Q. Obesity, allergy, and immunology. J Allergy Clin Immunol 2005;115:1102-4.

29) Bettencourt PE, Del Bono EA, Spiegelman D et al. Clinical utility of chest auscultation in common pulmonary diseases. Am J Respir Crit Care Med 1994;150:1291-7.

30) Beuther DA, Sutherland ER. Obesity and pulmonary function testing. J Allergy Clin Immunol 2005;115:1100-1.

31) Beuther DA, Weiss ST, Sutherland ER. Obesity and asthma. Am J Respir Crit Care Med 2006;17:112-9.

32) Beveridge RC, Grunfeld AF, Hodder RV et al. Guidelines for the emergency management of asthma in adults. CAEP/CTS Asthma Advisory Committee. Canadian Association of Emergency Physicians and the Canadian Thoracic Society. CMAJ 1996;155:25-37.

33) Bogaert D, van der Valk P, Ramdin R et al. Host-pathogen interaction during pneumococcal infection in patients with chronic obstructive pulmonary disease. Infect Immun 2004;72:818-823.

34) Bone RC, Boyars M, Braun SR et al. In chronic obstructive pulmonary disease, a combination of ipratropium and albuterol is more effective than either agent alone: an 85-day multicenter trial. Chest 1994;105:1411-9.

35) Bonomo RA. Resistant pathogens in respiratory tract infections in older people. J Am Geriatr Soc 2002;S236-41.

36) Boulet LP, Chapman KR. Asthma Education: The Canadian Experience. Chest 1994;106:206S-210.

37) Boulet LP, Becker A, Bérubé D et al. Canadian Asthma Consensus Report, 1999. Canadian Asthma Consensus Group. CMAJ 1999;161:S1-61.

38) Boulet LP, Bai T, Becker A et al. What is new since the last (1999) Canadian Asthma Consensus Guidelines? Can Respir J 2001;8:5A-27.

39) Bourbeau J, Rouleau M, Boucher S. A double blind randomized study of inhaled budesonide in patients with steroid responsive COPD. Am Rev Respir Dis 1994;147:A317.

40) Bourbeau J, Rouleau M, Boucher S. Randomized, controlled trial of inhaled corticosteroids in patients with chronic obstructive pulmonary disease. Thorax 1998;53: 477-82.

41) Bourbeau J, Julien M, Maltais F et al. Reduction of hospital utilization in patients with chronic pulmonary disease: A disease-specific self-management intervention. Arch Intern Med 2003;163:585-91.

42) Bourbeau J, Nault D, Dang-Tan T. Self-management and behaviour modification in COPD. Patient Educ Couns 2004;53:271- 7.

43) Boyd G, Morice AH, Pounsford JC et al. An evaluation of salmeterol in the treatment of chronic obstructive pulmonary disease (COPD). Eur Respir J 1997;10:815-21.

44) Bracken MB, Triche EW, Belanger K et al. Asthma symptoms, severity, and drug therapy: a prospective study of effects on 2205 pregnancies. Obstet Gynecol 2003;102:739-52.

45) Braun SR, McKenzie WN, Copeland C et al. A comparison of the effect of Ipratropium and Albuterol in the treatment of chronic obstructive airway disease. Arch Intern Med 1989;149:544-7.

46) Brisbon N, Plumb J, Brawer R et al. The asthma and obesity epidemics: The role played by the built environment – a public health perspective. J Allergy Clin Immunol 2005;115:1024-8.

47) BTS (British Thoracic Society / NICE). BTS: Chronic Obstructive Pulmonary Disease. National clinical guideline on management of chronic obstructive pulmonary disease in primary and secondary care. Thorax 2004;59:1-232.

48) BTS (British Thoracic Society) BTS: Guideline on the management of asthma: a national clinical guideline. British Thoracic Society/Scottish Intercollegiate Guidelines Network: London; 2005. Available at http://www.brit-thoracic.org.uk.

49) Brussee JE, Smit HA, van Strein RT et al. Allergen exposure in infancy and the development of sensitization, wheeze, and asthma at 4 years. J Allergy Clin Immunol 2005;115:946-52.

50) Buist AS. Risk Factors for COPD. Eur Respir Rev 1996;6:253-8.

51) Burge PS, Calverley PMA, Jones PW et al. Randomised, double blind, placebo controlled study of fluticasone propionate in patients with moderate to severe chronic obstructive disease: the ISOLDE trial. BMJ 2000;320: 1297-303.

52) Busse W, Nelson H, Wolfe J, Kalberg C, Yancey SW, Rickard KA. Comparison of inhaled salmeterol and oral zafirlukast in patients with asthma. J Allergy Clin Immunol 1999;103:1075-80.

53) Butler J, Breiman R, Campbell J et al. Pneomococcal polysaccharide vaccine efficacy: an evalution of current recommendations. JAMA 1993;270:1826-31.

54) Callahan CM, Dittus RS, Katz BP. Oral corticosteroid therapy for patients with stable chronic obstructive pulmonary disease. A meta-analysis. Ann Int Med 1991;114:216-23.

55) Calverley PM, Anderson JA, Celli B et al. Salmeterol and fluticasone propionate and survival in chronic obstructive pulmonary disease. N Engl J Med 2007;356:775-89.

56) Calverley PM, Boonsawat W, Cseke Z et al. Maintenance therapy with budesonide and formoterol in chronic obstructive pulmonary disease. Eur Respir J 2003;22:912-9.

57) Canadian Immunization Guide. 6th Edition. Health Canada: Ottawa. 2002.

58) CIHI (Canadian Institute for Health Information) and Canadian Lung Association. Respiratory Disease in Canada. Health Canada: Ottawa. 2001.

59) CTS (Canadian Thoracic Society) Workshop Group. Guidelines for the assessment and management of chronic obstructive pulmonary disease. Can Med Assoc J 1992;147:420-8.

60) Castro-Rodríguez J, Holberg C, Wright A, et al. A clinical index to define risk of asthma in young children with recurrent wheezing. Am J Respir Crit Care Med 2000;162;1403-6.

61) CCS/NCIC (Canadian Cancer Society/National Cancer Institute of Canada): Canadian Cancer Statistics 2006, Toronto, Canada, 2006.

62) Celedon JC, Litonjua AA, Ryan L, et al. Exposure to cat allergen, maternal history of asthma, and wheezing in first 5 years of life. Lancet 2002;360:781-2.

63) Celli BR, Cote CG, Martin JM et al. The body-mass index, airflow obstruction, dyspnea, and exercise capacity index in chronic obstructive pulmonary disease. N Eng J Med 2004;350:1005-12.

64) Celli BR, MacNee W; ATS/ERS Task Force. Standards for the diagnosis and treatment of patients with COPD: a summary of the ATS/ERS position paper. Eur Respir J. 2004;23:932-46.

65) Celli BR, Snider GL, Heffner J et al. American Thoracic Society. Standards for the diagnosis and care of patients with chronic obstructive pulmonary disease. Am J Respir Crit Care Med 1995;152:S77-120.

66) Chalmers GW, Macleod KJ, Little SA et al. Influence of cigarette smoking on inhaled corticosteroid treatment in mild asthma. Thorax 2002;57:226-30.

67) Chan B, Anderson G, Dales RE. Spirometry utilization in Ontario: practice patterns and policy implications. Can Med Assoc J 1997;156:169-76.

68) Chapman KR. Therapeutic approaches to chronic obstructive pulmonary disease: an emerging consensus. Am J Med 1996;100:5S-10.

69) Chapman KR, Mannino DM, Soriano JB et al. Epidemiology and costs of chronic obstructive pulmonary disease. Eur Respir J 2006;27:188-207.

70) Chaudhuri R, Livingston E, McMahon AD et al. Cigarette smoking impairs the therapeutic response to oral corticosteroids in chronic asthma. Am J Respir Crit Care Med 2003;168:1308-11.

71) Chaudhuri R, Livingston E, McMahon AD et al. Effects of smoking cessation on lung function and airway inflammation in smokers with asthma. Am J Respir Crit Care Med 2006;174:127-33.

72) Chen DK, McGeer A, de Azavedo JC et al. Decreased susceptibility of Streptococcus pneumoniae to fluoroquinolones in Canada. Canadian Bacterial Surveillance Network. N Engl J Med 1999;341:233-9.

73) Cheung D, van Klink HC, Aalbers R, for the OZON study group. Improved lung function and symptom control with formoterol on demand in asthma. Eur Respir J 2006;27:504-10.

74) Chroinin MNi, Greenstone IR, Danish A et al. Lon-acting β_2-agonists versus placebo in addition to inhaled corticosteroids in children and adults with chronic asthma. Cochrane Database of Syst Rev 2005;CD005535.

75) Clay KD, Hanson, JS, Pope SD, et al. Brief Communication: Severe hepatotoxicity of telithromycin: Three case reports and literature review. Ann Intern Med 2006; 44: 415-20.

76) Creticos PS. The consideration of immunotherapy in the treatment of allergic asthma. J Allergy Clin Immunol 2000;105:S559-74.

77) Curtis JR, Martin DP, Martine TR. Patient-assessed health outcomes in chronic lung disease. Am J Respir Crit Care Med 1997;156:1032-9.

78) Davies L, Angus RM, Calverley PM. Oral corticosteroids in patients admitted to hospital with exacerbations of chronic obstructive pulmonary disease: a prospective, randomized controlled trial. Lancet 1999;354:456-60.

79) Day A, Singer L. Pulmonary Medicine: Lessons in women's health. Ontario Thoracic Reviews. Summer 1998,10:1-7.

80) Derom E, Van De Velde V, Marissens S, et al. Effects of inhaled ciclesonide and fluticasone propionate on cortisol secretion and airway responsiveness to adenosine 5' monophosphate in asthmatic patients. Pulmonary Pharmacology & Therapeutics 2005;18:328-36.

81) Devereux G, Seaton A. Diet as a risk factor for atopy and asthma. J Allergy Clin Immunol 2005;115:1109-17.

82) Devine EC, Rearcy J. Meta-analysis of the effects of psycho educational care in adults with chronic obstructive pulmonary disease. Patient Educ Couns 1996;29:167-78.

83) Dolovich MB, Ahrens RC, Hess DR et al. Device selection and outcomes of aerosol therapy: Evidence-based guidelines. Chest 2005;127:335-71.

84) Donohue JF, van Noord JA, Bateman ED et al. A 6-month, placebo-controlled study comparing lung function and health status changes in COPD patients treated with tiotropium or salmeterol. Chest 2002;122:47-55.

85) D'Urzo AD, Chapman KR. Leukotriene-receptor antagonists. Role in asthma management. Can Fam Physician 2000;46:872-9.

86) Emerman CL, Connors AF, Lukens TW et al. A randomized controlled trial of methylprednisólone in the emergency treatment of acute exacerbations of COPD. Chest 1989;95:563-7.

87) Ernst P, McIvor A, Ducharme FM et al. Safety and effectiveness of long acting inhaled β_2-agonist bronchodilators when taken with inhaled corticosteroids. Ann Intern Med 2006;145:692-4.

88) Etter J, Stapelton JA. Nicotine replacement therapy for long-term smoking cessation: a meta-analysis. Tob Control 2006;15:280-5.

89) Fantuzzi G. Adipose tissue, adipokines, and inflammation. J Allergy Clin Immunol 2005;115:911-9.

90) Ferguson GT, Cherniack RM. Management of chronic obstructive pulmonary disease. N Engl J Med 1993 Apr;328:1017-22.

91) Fletcher CM, Elmes PC, Wood CH. The significance of respiratory symptoms and the diagnosis of chronic bronchitis in a working population. Br Med J 1959;1:257-66.

92) Fletcher CM, Peto R. The national history of chronic airflow obstruction. BMJ 1977; 1:1645-8.

93) Ford ES. The epidemiology of obesity and asthma. J Allergy Clin Immunol 2005;115:897-909.

94) Friedman NJ, Zeiger RS. The role of breast-feeding in the development of allergies and asthma. J Allergy Clin Immunol 2005;115:1238-48.

95) Gartlehner G, Hansen R, Carson S et al. Efficacy and safety of inhaled corticosteroids in patient with COPD: A systematic review and meta-analysis of health outcomes. Ann Fam Med 2006;4:253-262.

96) Gern JE, Reardon CL, Hoffjan S et al. Effects of dog ownership and genotype on immune development and atopy in infancy. J Allergy Clin Immunol 2004;113:307-14.

97) Gibson PG, Henry RL, Coughlan JL. Gastro-oesophageal reflux treatment for asthma in adults and children. Cochrane Database Sys Rev 2003;(2):CD001496.

98) GINA (Global Initiative for Asthma). Global strategy for asthma management and prevention: A practical guide for public health care professionals. 2006. Available at: http://www.ginasthma.com.

99) Glenny RW. Steroids in COPD. The scripture according to Albert. Chest 1987;91:289-90.

100) GOLD (Global Initiative for Chronic Obstructive Lung Disease). Global strategy for the diagnosis, management, and prevention of chronic obstructive pulmonary disease. 2006. Available at: http://www.goldcopd.org.

101) Gold DR, Wang X, Wypij D et al. Effects of cigarette smoking on lung function in adolescent boys and girls. N Engl J Med 1996;335:931-7.

102) Greenstone IR, Chroinin Ni, Masse V et al. Combination of long-acting β_2-agonists and inhaled steroids versus higher dose of inhaled steroids in children and adults with persistent asthma. Cochrane Database Sys Rev 2005;CD005533.

103) Grossman RF. The value of antibiotics and the outcomes of antibiotic therapy in exacerbations of COPD. Chest 1998;113:249S-255.

104) Grossman RF. Guidelines for the treatment of acute exacerbations of chronic bronchitis. Chest 1997;112:310S-313.

105) Grossman RF, Mukherjee J, Vaughan D et al. A 1-year community-based health economic study of ciprofloxacin vs usual antibiotic treatment in acute exacerbations of chronic bronchitis: the Canadian Ciprofloxacin Health Economic Study Group. Chest 1998;113:131-41.

106) Hansen-Flaschen J. COPD: The Last Year of Life. Respir Care 2004;49:90-7.

107) Health Canada Advisory – Safety information about a class of asthma drugs known as long-acting-beta2-agonists. Health Canada. October 4, 2005.

108) Health Canada Advisory – Antibiotic Ketek and possible association with liver failure. Health Canada. February 7, 2006.

109) Health Canada Advisory - Updated safety information on KETEK (telithromycin) and hepatic events, aggravation of myasthenia gravis and syncope. Ottawa. September 29, 2006.

110) Hughes JR, Stead LF, Lancaster T. Antidepressants for smoking cessation. Cochrane Database of Syst Rev 2004;CD000031.

111) ICES (Institute for Clinical Evaluative Sciences). To T, Gershon A, Tassoudji M, et al. The burden of asthma in Onatrio. Toronto: September 2006.

112) Ikeda A, Nishimura K, Koyama H et al. Bronchodilating effects of combined therapy with clinical dosages of ipratropium bromide and salbutamol for stable COPD: comparison with ipratropium bromide alone. Chest 1995;107:401-5.

113) ICSI (Institute for Clinical Systems Improvement). Health Care Guideline: Diagnosis and Outpatients Management of Asthma. NQMC 2005;001717-20.

114) IPAG (International Primary Care Airways Group). Chronic airways diseases: a guide for primary care physicians. MCR VISION, Inc., 2005.

115) Jarjour NN, Wilson SJ, Koenig SM et al. Control of airway inflammation maintained at a lower syeroid dose with 100/50 µg of fluticasone propionate/salmeterol. J Allergy Clin Immunol 2006;118:44-52.

116) Johnson CC, Ownby DR, Alford SH et al. Antibiotic exposure in early infancy and risk for childhood atopy. J Allergy Clin Immunol 2005;115:1218-24.

117) Johnston NW, Sears MR. A national evaluation of geographic and temporal patterns of hospitalization of children for asthma in Canada [abstract]. Am J Respir Crit Care Med 2001;163:A359.

118) Johnston NW, Johnston SL, Duncan JM et al. The September epidemic of asthma exacerbations in children: a search for etiology. J Allergy Clin Immunol. 2005;115:132-8 and 230-2.

119) Kelsen SG, Church NL, Gillman SA et al. Salmeterol added to inhaled corticosteroid therapy is superior to doubling the dose of inhaled corticosteroids: a randomized clinical trial. J Asthma 1999;36:703-15.

120) Klassen L. Opening the airways. Pharmacy Practice 1998;14:45-59.

121) Krahn MD, Berka C, Langlois P et al. Direct and indirect costs of asthma in Canada, 1990. CMAJ 1996;154:821-31.

122) Larabie LC. To what extext do smokers plan quit attempts? Tobacco Control 2005;14:425-8.

123) Lacasse Y, Guyatt GH, Goldstein RS. The components of a respiratory rehabilitation program: a systematic review. Chest 1997;111:1077-88.

124) Lacasse Y, Brooks D, Goldstein RS. Trends in the epidemiology of COPD in Canada, 1980-1995. Presented at the ALA/ATS 1998 International Conference. Chicago. April 24-29th, 1998.

125) Lemière C, Bai T, Balter M et al. Adult asthma consensus guidelines update 2003. Can Respir J 2004;11:9A-18.

126) Lofdahl CG, Reiss TF, Leff JA et al. Randomized, placebo controlled trial of effect of a leukotriene receptor antagonist, montelukast, on tapering inhaled corticosteroids in asthmatic patients. BMJ 1999;319:87-90.

127) Lokke A, Lange P, Scharling H et al. Developing COPD: a 25 year follow up study of the general population. Thorax 2006;61:935-9.

128) Lowry JB. A Guide to Spirometry for Primary Care Physicians 1998. Published by Boehringer Ingelheim. Endorsed by the College of Family Physicians of Canada and the Canadian Thoracic Society.

129) Lucas SR and Platts-Mills TAE. Physical activity and exercise in asthma: Relevance to etiology and treatment. J Allergy Clin Immunol 2005;115:928-34.

130) Luskin AT. An overview of the recommendations of the Working Group on Asthma and Pregnancy. National Asthma Education and Prevention Program. J Allergy Clin Immunol 1999;103:S350-3.

131) Mahler DA, Tomlinson D, Olmstead EM et al. Changes in dyspnea, health status, and lung function in chronic airway disease. Am J Respir Crit Care Med 1995;151:61-5.

132) Mahler DA, Wells CK. Evaluation of clinical methods for rating dyspnea. Chest 1998;93:580-6.

133) Mao Y, Semenciw R, Morrison H et al. Increased Rates of Illness and Death from Asthma in Canada. CMAJ 1987;137:620-4.

134) Marcus P. Incorporating anti-IgE (omalizumab) therapy into pulmonary medicine practice: practice management implications. Chest 2006;129:466-74.

135) Marra F, Lynd L, Coombes M et al. Does antibiotic exposure during infancy lead to development of asthma?: a systematic review and metaanalysis. Chest 2006;129:610-8.

136) Martinez FD, Wright AL, Taussig LM, et al. Asthma and wheezing in the first six years of life. N Engl J Med 1995;332:133-8.

137) McFadden RG, Marshall BE. Antibiotic therapy in COPD. Hosp Formul 1992;27:595-607.

138) Melen E, Wickman M, Nordvall SL et al. Influence of early and current environmental exposure factors on sensitization and outcome of asthma in pre-school children. Allergy 2001;56:646-52.

139) Morbidity and Mortality Weekly Report (MMWR). Recommendations of the immunization practices advisory committee pneumococcal polysaccharide vaccine. MMWR Weekly 1989;38:64-68, 73-76.

140) Miyamoto K, Aida A, Nishimura M et al. Gender effect on prognosis of patients receiving long-term home oxygen therapy. The Respiratory Failure Research Group in Japan. Am J Respir Crit Care Med 1995;152:972-6.

141) Murata GH, Gorby MS, Chick TW et al. Intravenous and oral corticosteroids for the prevention of relapse after treatment of decompensated COPD. Effect on patient with a history of multiple relapses. Chest 1990;98:845-9.

142) Murphy TF, Sethi S. Bacterial infection in chronic obstructive pulmonary disease. Am Rev Respir Dis 1992;146:1067-83.

143) NACTF (National Asthma Control Task Force). The Prevention and Management of Asthma in Canada: A Major Challenge Now and in the Future. Ottawa: The National Asthma Control Task Force – Health Canada: Ottawa. 2000.

144) NAEPP (National Asthma Education and Prevention Program). Expert Panel Report 2 – Guidelines for the Diagnosis and Management of Asthma. National Institutes of Health – National Heart, Lung, and Blood Institute. Publication No. 97 – 4051. Available at: http://www.nhlbi.nih.gov/guidelines/asthma/asthgdln.htm. 1997 and 2002 and 2004 updates.

145) Naganathan V, Jones G, Nash P et al. Vertebral fracture risk with long-term corticosteroid therapy: prevalence and relation to age, bone density, and corticosteroid use. Arch Intern Med 2000;160:2917-22.

146) Nelson HS. Long-acting β_2-agonists in adult asthma: evidence that these drugs are safe. Prim Care Resp J 2006;15:271-7.

147) Nelsen LP, Pederesen B, Faurschou P et al. Salmeterol reduces the need for inhaled corticosteroid in steroid-dependent asthmatics. Respir Med 1999;93:863-8.

148) Newman Taylor AJ and Nicholson PJ (Eds.). Guidelines for the prevention, identification and management of occupational asthma: Evidence review and recommendations. British Occupational Health Research Foundation. London. 2004.

149) Nicholson PJ, Cullinan P, Newman Taylor AJ et al. Evidence based guidelines for the prevention, identification and management of occupational asthma. Occup Environ Med 2005;62:290-9.

150) Niewoehner DE, Erbland ML, Deupree RH et al. Effect of systemic glucocorticoids on exacerbations of chronic obstructive pulmonary disease. N Engl J Med 1999;340:1941-7.

151) NIH (National Institutes of Health) State-of-the-Science conference statement: tobacco use: prevention, cessation, and control. Ann Intern Med. 2006;145:839-44.

152) Nishimura K, Izumi T, Tsukino M et al, Dyspnea is a better predictor of 5-year survival than airway obstruction in patients with COPD. Chest 2002;121:1434-40.

153) O'Byrne PM, Bisgaard H, Godard PP, et al. Budesonide/Formoterol combination therapy as both maintenance and reliever medication in asthma. Am J Respir Crit Care Med 2005;171:129-36.

154) O'Byrne PM, Pedersen S, Busse WW et al. Effects of early intervention with inhaled budesonide on lung function in newly diagnosed asthma. CHEST 2006;129:1478-85.

155) O'Donnell DE, Aaron S, Bourbeau J et al. Canadian Thoracic Society recommendations for management of chronic obstructive pulmonary disease 2003. Can Respir J 2003;10:11A-65.

156) O'Donnell DE, Aaron S, Bourbeau J et al. State of the Art Compendium: Canadian Thoracic Society recommendations for the management of chronic obstructive pulmonary disease. Can Respir J 2004;11:7B-59.

157) O'Donnell DE, Fluge T, Gerken F et al. Effects of tiotropium on lung hyperinflation, dyspnoea and exercise tolerance in COPD. Eur Respir J 2004;23:832-840.

158) O'Donnell DE, Sciurba F, Celli b et al. Effect of Fluticasone Propionate/Salmeterol on Lung Hyperinflation and Exercise Endurance in COPD. Chest 2006;130:647-56.

159) Ownby DR, Johnson CC, Peterson EL. Exposure to dogs and cats in the first year of life and risk of allergic sensitization at 6 to 7 years of age. JAMA 2002;288:963-72.

160) Pedersen B, Dahl R, Karlstrom R et al. Eosinophil and neutrophil activity in asthma in a one-year trial with inhaled budesonide. The impact of smoking. Am J Respir Crit Care Med 1996;153:1519-29.

161) Physician Consortium for Performance Improvement. Clinical performance measures: Asthma. American Medical Association: AP25:03-0261:1.7M:7/03. Available at: www.ama-assn.org/go/quality.

162) Platts-Mills T, Vaughan J, Squillace S et al. Sensitisation, asthma, and a modified Th2 response in children exposed to cat allergen: a population-based cross-sectional study. Lancet 2001;357:752-6.

163) Prodigy Guidance. Asthma. London: NHS – National Library of Health; 2006.

164) Prodigy Guidance. COPD. London: NHS – National Library of Health; 2006.

165) Product Monograph Update. Ketek (Telithromycin); Health Canada endorsed important safety information on Ketek. Sanofi-Aventis; September 29, 2006.

166) Rabe KF. Treating COPD - the TORCH trial, P values, and the dodo. N Engl J Med 2007;356:851-4.

167) Rabe KF, Pizzichini E, Stallberg B, et al. Budesonide/Formoterol in a single inhaler for maintenance and relief in mild-to-moderate asthma. Chest 2006; 129: 246-56.

168) Rabe KF, Atienza T, Magyar P, et al. Effect of budesonide in combination with formoterol for reliever therapy in asthma exacerbations: a randomised controlled, double-blind study. Lancet 2006a; 368: 744-53.

169) Ranney L, Melvin C, Lux L et al. Systematic review: smoking cessation intervention strategies for adults and adults in special populations. Ann Intern Med 2006;145;845-56.

170) Rey E, Boulet LP. Asthma in pregnancy. BMJ 2007;334:582-5.

171) Risch HA, Howe GR, Jain M et al. Lung cancer risk for female smokers. Science 1994;263:1206-8.

172) Rodrigo G, Rodrigo C, Burschin O. A meta-analysis of the effect of ipratropium bromide in adults with acute asthma. Am J Med 1999;107:363-70.

173) Rosser WW, Pennie RA, Pilla NJ and the Anti-infective Review Panel. Anti-infective guidelines for community-acquired infections. Toronto: MUMS Guideline Clearinghouse;2005.

174) Ruigómez A, Rodríguez LA, Wallander M et al. Gastroesophageal reflux disease and asthma: a longitudinal study in UK practice. Chest 2005;128:85-93.

175) Rutten-Van Molken MP, Van Doorslae EK, Jansen MC et al. Costs and effects of inhaled corticosteroids and bronchodilators in asthma and chronic obstructive pulmonary disease. Am J Respir Crit Care Med 1995;151: 975-82.

176) Saint S, Bent S, Vittinghoff E et al. Antibiotics in chronic obstructive pulmonary disease exacerbations. A meta-analysis. JAMA 1995;273:957-60.

177) Salpeter SR, Buckley NS, Ormiston TM et al. Meta-analysis: effect of long-acting β_2-agonists on severe asthma exacerbations and asthma-related deaths. Ann Intern Med 2006;144:904-12.

178) Sethi S, Evans N, Grant BJ et al. New strains of bacteria and exacerbations of chronic obstructive pulmonary disease. N Engl J Med 2002;347:465-71.

179) Sharek PJ, Bergman DA, Ducharme F. Beclomethasone for asthma in children: effects on linear growth. Cochrane Database Syst Rev 1999;CD001282.

180) Sheikh A, Alves B, Dhami S. Pneumococcal vaccine for asthma. Cochrane Database Syst Rev 2002;CD002165. Updated August 2004.

181) Shim CS, Williams MH Jr. Aerosol beclomethasone in patients with steroid-responsive chronic obstructive pulmonary disease. Am J Med 1985;78:655-8.

182) Shore SA, Fredberg JJ. Obesity, smooth muscle, and hyperresponsiveness. J Allergy Clin Immunol 2005;115:925-7.

183) Siafakas NM, Vermeire P, Pride NB et al. Optimal assessment and management of chronic obstructive pulmonary disease (COPD): The European Respiratory Society Task Force. Eur Respir J 1995;8:1398-420.

184) Silagy C, Lancaster T, Stead L et al. Nicotine replacement therapy for smoking cessation. Cochrane Database Syst Rev 2004;CD000146.

185) (SMART trial) Nelson HS, Scott TW, Bleecker ER, et al. The salmeterol multicenter asthma research trial (SMART):A comparison of usual pharmacotherapy for asthma or usual pharmacotherapy plus salmeterol. Chest 2006;129:15-26.

186) Snow V, Lascher S, Mottur-Pilson C. Evidence base for management of acute exacerbations of chronic obstructive pulmonary disease. Ann Intern Med 2001;134:595-9.

187) Sood A. Does obesity weigh heavily on the health of the human airway? J Allergy Clin Immunol 2005;115:921-4.

188) Stockley RA, O'Brien C, Pye A et al. Relationship of sputum colour to nature and outpatient management of acute exacerbations of COPD. Chest 2000;117:1638-45.

189) Stoodley RG, Aaron SD, Dales RE. The role of ipratropium bromide in the emergency management of acute asthma exacerbation: a metaanalysis of randomized clinical trials. Ann Emerg Med 1999;34:8-18.

190) Stubbing DG, Mathur PN, Roberts RS et al. Some physical signs in patients with chronic airflow obstruction. Am Rev Respir Dis 1982;125:549-52.

191) Szafranski W, Cukier A, Ramirez A et al. Efficacy and safety of budesonide/formoterol in the management of chronic obstructive pulmonary disease. Eur Respir J 2003;21:74-81.

192) Tarlo S. Cough: Occupational and environmental considerations - ACCP evidence-based clinical practice guidelines. Chest 2006;129:186S-196S.

193) Tarlo SM, Boulet LP, Cartier A et al. Canadian Thoracic Society Guidelines for occupational asthma. Can Respir J 1998;5:289-300.

194) Tarlo SM, Liss GM. Occupational asthma: An approach to diagnosis and management. CMAJ 2003;168:867-71.

195) Tattersfield AE, Lofdahl CG, Postma DS et al. Comparison of formoterol and terbutaline for as-needed treatment of asthma: a randomised trial. Lancet 2001;357:257-61.

196) Terzano C, Petroianni A, Ricci A et al. Combination therapy in COPD: different response of COPD stages and predictivity of functional parameters. Eur Rev Med Pharmacol Sci 2005;9:209-15.

197) The Childhood Asthma Management Program Research Group. Long-term effects of budesonide or nedocromil in children with asthma. N Engl J Med 2000;343:1054-63.

198) Thompson WH, Nielson CP, Carvalho P et al. Controlled trial of oral prednisone in outpatients with acute COPD exacerbation. Am J Respir Crit Care Med 1996;154:407-12.

199) U.S. Public Health Service report. The Tobacco Use and Dependence Clinical Practice Guideline Panel, Staff, and Consortium Representatives. A clinical practice guideline for treating tobacco use and dependence. JAMA 2000;283:3244-54.

200) van der Meer RM, Wagena EJ, Ostelo RWJG et al. Smoking cessation for chronic obstructive pulmonary disease. Cochrane Database Syst Rev 2001;CD002999.

201) Vogelmeier C, D'Urzo A, Pauwels R. Budesonide/Formoterol maintenance and reliever therapy: an effective asthma treatment option? Eur Respir J 2005;26:819-28.

202) Walters JAE, Walters EH, Wood-Baker R. Oral corticosteroids for stable chronic obstructive pulmonary disease. Cochrane Database Syst Rev 2005;CD005374.

203) Wang J, Visness CM, Sampson HA. Food allergen sensitization in inner-city children with asthma. J Allergy Clin Immunol 2005;115:1076-80.

204) Ward KD, Klesges RC, Zbikowski SM et al. Gender differences in the outcome of an unaided smoking cessation attempt. Addict Behav 1997;22:521-33.

205) West R, Sohal T. "Catastrophic" pathways to smoking cessation:findings from national survey. BMJ 2006;332:458-60.

206) Wilson JD, Serby CW, Menjoge SS et al. The efficacy and safety of combination bronchodilator therapy. Eur Respir Rev 1996;6:286-9.

207) Wilson R, Schentag J, Ball P et al. A comparison of gemifloxacin and clarithromycin in acute exacerbations of chronic bronchitis and long-term clinical outcomes. Clin Ther 2002;24:639-52.

208) Wilson R, Allegra L, Huchon G et al. Short-term and long-term outcomes of moxifloxacin compared to standard antibiotic treatment in acute exacerbations of chronic bronchitis. Chest 2004;125:953-64.

209) Woolcock NJ, Ollerenshaw S. Studies of airway inflammation in asthma and chronic airflow limitation. Do they help to explain cause? Am J Respir Crit Care Med 1994;150:S103-5.

210) Zervos MJ, Heyder AM, Leroy B. Oral telithromycin 800mg once daily for 5 days cersus cefuroxime axetil 500mg twice daily for 10 days in adults with acute exacerbations of chronic bronchitis. J Int Med Res 2003;31:157-69.

211) Zhanel GG, Walters M, Noreddin A et al. The ketolides: A critical review. Drugs 2002;62:1771-804.

General Comment Sheet

We appreciate any suggestions and recommendations you may have. Please note any extensive comments on the back of this form or directly on the specific page. You may also submit an online form from our website, which is available at:

www.mumshealth.com/content/order_forms/guideline_comment_sheet.pdf

Item		Comments
1. Is this guideline concise, easy to understand?	❏ Yes ❏ No	
2. Would you recommend any content changes?	❏ Yes ❏ No	
3. Would you recommend any format changes?	❏ Yes ❏ No	
4. How often do you refer to guidelines in your practice?	❏ Daily ❏ Weekly ❏ Monthly ❏ Rarely	
5. (a) Which specific guideline(s) do you refer to most often? (b) Why?		

To assure accurate acknowledgment in the guidelines as an external reviewer, please provide the following information:

Name: _____   Type of Practice: _____

Affiliation (if applicable): _____

City/Town: _____   Province: _____

Phone: _____   Fax: _____   Email: _____

Please return to:

MUMS Guideline Clearinghouse, **#901 – 790 Bay St., Toronto, Ontario M5G 1N8 or fax (416) 597-8574 or e-mail: guidelines@mumshealth.com**